OUT OF SIGHT INTO VISION

OUT OF SIGHT
INTO VISION

There is more to good vision
than reading the fine print.

Neville S. Cohen, O.D.
Joseph L. Shapiro, O.D.

SIMON AND SCHUSTER   NEW YORK

Copyright© 1977 by Collier Macmillan Canada, Ltd.

Published by Simon and Schuster
A Division of Gulf & Western Corporation
Simon & Schuster Building
Rockefeller Center
1230 Avenue of the Americas
New York, New York 10020

Designed by Brant Cowie/Artplus, Toronto
Illustrations by Joan Affleck, Toronto
Photographs by Brenda Halpern, Brooklyn, New York
Cover photograph by Paterson Photographic Works, Toronto
Manufactured in the United States of America
1 2 3 4 5 6 7 8 9 10

Library of Congress Cataloging in Publication Data

Cohen, Neville S, date.
  Out of sight into vision.

  Includes index.
  1. Vision disorders. 2. Vision. I. Shapiro,
Joseph L., date, joint author. II. Title.
RE51.C63 1977   617.7'5   77-7603
ISBN 0-671-22940-0

This book is for all those
who want a better understanding
of their vision.
An informed public
is an aware public;
an aware public asks questions.

CONTENTS

ACKNOWLEDGMENTS

The major concepts for this book were laid down by the Optometric Extension Program, the Gesell Institute of Child Development, and the University Optometric Center, an affiliated clinical institution of the State College of Optometry, State University of New York.

Grateful acknowledgment is specifically due to the following for permitting us to use material and quote selected excerpts from the works cited:

Bartlett, J.D., *Isometropic Meridional Aniseikonia:* A Case Report. Journal of the American Optometric Association, February 1975.

Birnbaum, Martin H., *Gross Motor and Postural Characteristics of Strabismus Patients.* Journal of the American Optometric Association, June 1974.

Birnbaum, Martin H. and I. Greenwald, *Orthoptics and Visual Training.* Journal of the American Optometric Association, Vol. 38, No. 12, December 1967.

Borish, I.M., *Clinical Refraction.* Chicago, Illinois: The Professional Press, Third Edition, 1970.

Eger, Milton J., *The Integrity of a Profession.* Journal of the American Optometric Association, October 1970.

Harmon, Darell Boyd, *The Coordinated Classroom.* Grand Rapids, Michigan: American Seating Company, 1953 by permission of the Darell Boyd Harmon Resource Center, Clayton, Missouri.

Notes on a Dynamic Theory of Vision. State College of Optometry © D. B. Harmon, 1958.

Kephart, Newell C. *The Slow Learner in the Classroom.* Columbus, Ohio: Charles E. Merrill Publishing Company, 1971.

Lowry, Raymond W. *The Free-Hand Square Test.* Handbook of Diagnostic Tests for the Developmental Optometrist. © R. W. Lowry, 1970.

Ludlam, William M. *Mr. F. F.'s Story—A Case History.* Journal of the American Optometric Association, May 1975.

Macdonald, Lawrence W. *Implications of Critical Empathy, Primal Scream and Identity Crisis in Optometric Visual Therapy.* Journal of the American Optometric Association, October 1972.

Clinical Optometric Technique. Duncan, Oklahoma: Optometric Extension Program Foundation, Inc. (International), 1962.

Orem, R.C. *Learning to See, Seeing to Learn.* Johnstown, Pa.: Mafex Associates Inc., 1971.

Roy, Raymond R. *Symptomatology of Binocular Stress.* Chicago, Illinois: The Optometric Weekly, The Professional Press.

The Role of Binocular Stress in the Post-Whiplash Syndrome. Berkeley, California: The American Journal of Optometry and the Archives of the American Academy of Optometry, Volume 38, November 1961.

Ross, Marjorie S. *Role Relationships—The Three O's.* Journal of the American Optometric Association, May 1974.

State College of Optometry, State University of New York. *Basic Sensory Movement Activities for Children* by Drs. E. Forrest and D. Fitzgerald, Infants' Vision Clinic of the University Optometric Center, New York.

Specific Home Guidance for Binocular Problems. Infants' Vision Clinic of the University Optometric Center, New York.

The authors wish to thank their dear friend Michael Corris for his invaluable assistance. We are especially grateful to Drs. Leon Hoffman and Allen H. Cohen for allowing us to use their "before and after" photographs of strabismic children; to Mr. George Adamson, General Manager of King Optical Company, Toronto, for his helpful suggestions, and to the American Optical Corporation and Bausch & Lomb, Canada, for permitting us to reproduce some of their excellent eye charts.

For their critical readings we would like to thank the following persons: Fred Bleck, Ph.D., Drs. Raymond Helfand, and Arnold Sherman. We are also indebted to Dr. Sherman for allowing us to take photographs in his optometric office.

We wish to thank Larry Dent for his foresight and confidence in us, and are extremely grateful to Lesley Wyle whose ideas and editorial assistance have been invaluable.

A special acknowledgment is due to the American Optometric Association for their continuous efforts to provide quality vision care.

Neville S. Cohen, O.D.
Joseph L. Shapiro, O.D.

FOREWORD

In today's world, where most people are hard put to cope with the stresses and strains of everyday life—at home and on the job—there is an increasing need for information and know-how that the layman can use himself to reduce the wear and tear on his bodily system. Having spent 40 years of my life studying the manifold physiologic aspects of stress, I realize the urgency of this need. In my various books, articles, lectures and contacts with people in general, I have tried, and am still trying, to teach them what I have learned so that they may better understand the mechanisms of stress.

The efforts that we investigative physicians make in trying to get our message across are being constantly outpaced by the rapid development in all fields, and especially by the challenge of adjustment to everchanging tasks, aspirations and possibilities.

Many books have been written for the lay public on how to acquire "better sight," often "without glasses," but never before has there been one that teaches so many facts, and explodes so many myths about ocular problems. There is no doubt that defective vision can be both the cause and the result of the stress of life.

Today, millions suffer from headaches, inability to express themselves, learning disabilities and so on, without knowing that they really are plagued by stress affecting individual bodily functions, very commonly their eyesight.

I like to speak about matters I can evaluate from personal experience and, to me, *Out of Sight into*

Vision fills a much-deplored gap in our understanding of stress. It offers a succinct explanation of the ocular manifestations of stress and provides readers with enough information to permit them to be their own physicians.

I can only hope that *Out of Sight into Vision* will meet with the success it deserves, not only with its readership but also by encouraging further scientific work along these lines.

Hans Selye, M.D., C.C.
Professor and Director of the
Institute of Experimental Medicine
and Surgery, University of Montreal.

INTRODUCTION

MANY of you reading this introduction have vision problems of which you are unaware, although you may have been told by your eye doctor that you have 20/20 sight and there is nothing wrong with your eyes.

YOU MAY HAVE BEEN MISLED!

The idea that 20/20* SIGHT can be equated with comfortable, efficient VISION has never been scientifically validated. Despite this, the majority of practicing eye doctors see their patients' achievement of clear distance sight as the ultimate goal of vision analysis. But 20/20 sight is only one aspect of total visual performance. Just as you should not blindly reach for a pair of glasses as the panacea for your visual ills, so you should not accept without question your eye doctor's rationale for treatment of those ills.

We would like to help you to better evaluate this treatment. We also hope you will learn something about the functioning of your own eyesight and how to assess your current visual status, through a series of simple tests. Therefore, this book is for everyone who

---

*Outside the United States and Canada, 20/20 is equivalent to 6/6.

1

desires a deeper understanding of vision and its problems, problems which show signs of spreading in epidemic-like fashion. An estimated seventy-five million American children are crippled with them; one hundred million adults and children wear the outward, visible signs—glasses.

Certain commercial interests take advantage of our consumer-oriented society by promoting neon-lit superstores, which issue eyeglass guarantees while they conduct "quickie" eye tests and deliver shoddy workmanship. As a result, irreparable damage may be done to your eyes and your health in general. Behind-the-scenes disputes among various eye care custodians are slowly strangling good vision practice. We shall expose some of the poor practices, and the motives behind them, as we feel that our present system must be transformed into one that is more responsive to people's real visual needs.

Vision is a total body process and does not exist in isolation. Faulty vision patterns often induce faulty postural patterns—head tilts, shoulder slumps, and curved spines—all possible consequences of inefficient visual performance. We also pay a high price for the luxury of having two eyes instead of one. Various bizarre symptoms may appear, often resulting in psychological, neurological, or physical problems. These symptoms may actually be the warning signs of chronic, two-eyed stress.

This is not a book about eye diseases—cataracts, glaucoma, tumors, etc.; it is about vision, our most dominant sensory-motor function. Your sight is a sensory process, concerned with how clearly you see the world. Your vision is the *interpretation* of eyesight and happens in the brain. It thus represents a higher mental function. For vision to emerge, you had to evolve through a certain hierarchy of movements in space at an early age; this evolution is the complete process of learning to see.

Recognizing the fact that vision is learned, and therefore trainable, is in accord with the most recent biological and psychological developments. This concept is embedded in our alternative approach to complete visual care. A functional, behavioral model of vision takes into account not only the nature of visual patterns but also how they arose and where they will lead to. We consider time as a determinant in the evolution of a particular visual status, while vision enhancement, problem prevention, and re-mediation are concepts that transcend traditional treatment.

A child is visually in danger every step of the way. If parents fail to provide the necessary visual stimuli, their children's total way of life may suffer; clumsiness, poor judgment, under-achievement in school, and a negative opinion of oneself may be possible consequences. Not only the well-informed parent but also the observant teacher can be instrumental in early detection of vision problems.

We cannot ignore the reality of our rapidly shrinking, visual environment which imposes stresses upon us, virtually unknown to primitive man. Our environment has shifted from distance to near vision, from the unrestricted to the restricted visual field, from free to confined space, from *detection* at distance to *interpretation* at near range. Lenses that provide 20/20 detection at distance may be totally inadequate for visual interpretation at close range. Prescribing different lenses for different visual demands forms the basis of a novel approach to vision care.

To understand the nature of our visual system, we must redesign that part of our environment that is used for near-centered activity. Furniture and lighting must be adapted to accommodate good visual and body functioning.

Vision is the mode of perception that can thrust us on to new levels of awareness. We shall present a twofold approach—physical and perceptual—to help you develop this awareness. To reach it we must cultivate the kind of consciousness that will encompass "sensible seeing." By gaining a proper outlook and a wholesome way of looking at the world, we can become more truly "in tune" with ourselves and the world around us.

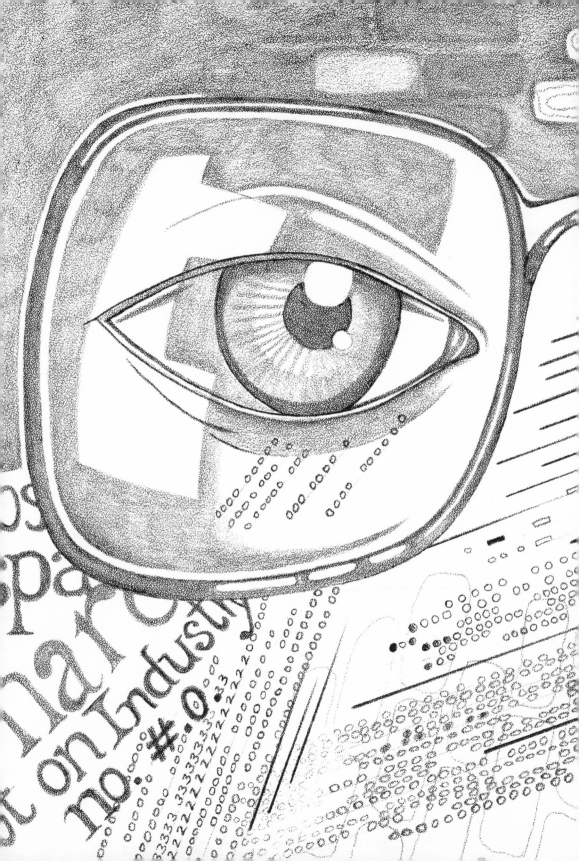

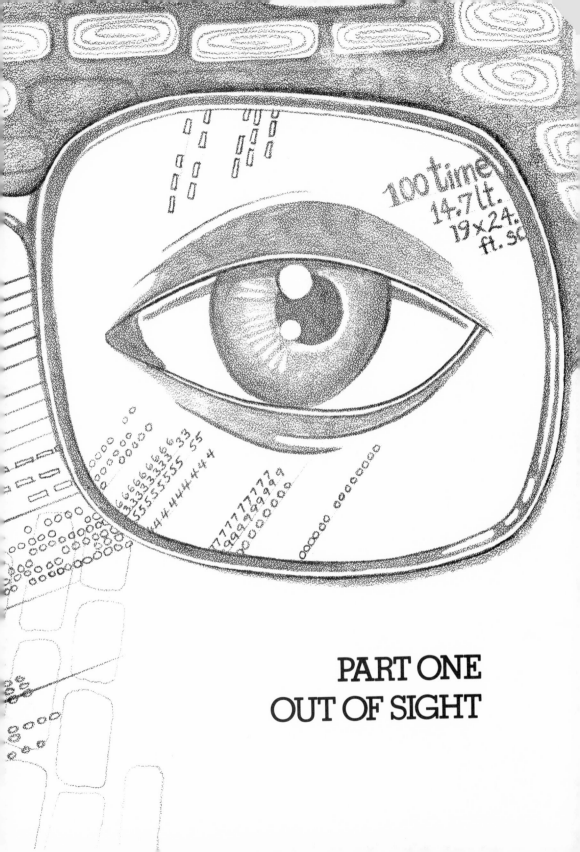

PART ONE
OUT OF SIGHT

CHAPTER ONE

LOOK OUT,
THE WORLD
IS CLOSING IN!

Do you think that the man who "sailed the seas" in his Yellow Submarine had 20/20 vision? And what about his friends who were with him? How well could they see? Pretty well, we suspect, when they first came aboard.

> In the town where I was born, lived a man who sailed the seas.
> And he told me of his life, in the land of submarines . . .
> We all live in a Yellow Submarine.
> *The Yellow Submarine*
> ©Maclen Music

But as they "sailed on to the sun," things began to change.

> The sky was not as blue nor the sea as green;
> Their vision got worse in that Yellow Submarine.
> And when our sailors, homeward bound,
> Stepped outside and looked around,
> They noticed a change most profound.

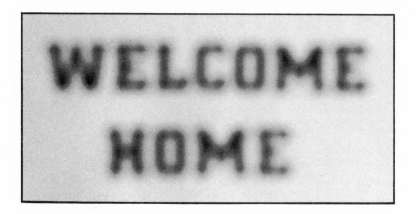

Not only their greeting sign, but everything off in the distance, looked blurred to them. During their physicals, a startling discovery was made: many of the sailors had lost the ability to see clearly at a distance!* Some of them also showed a tendency to turn their eyes inward towards their noses, a clinical sign of visual stress. It seemed as if in this man-made environment, these submarine sailors had been forced to "focus in" instead of "focusing out." What was it about their environment that could have caused this loss of distance vision? A submarine is a "shut-in" world, an environment with firmly imposed physical and visual restraints. (An actual study done in the United States has revealed a significant deterioration in submarine sailors' distance vision). Think of tall buildings in the core of any large city where distance viewing is as impossible as in a submarine. Then

---

*To check your distance vision, use the eye chart on inside jacket.

think about the desk in your room, the one pushed against the wall; does it allow you relaxed distance viewing?

In a submarine, in a schoolroom and in an office, vision is probably restricted to 10 feet (3 m) or less; most work is performed at a distance of perhaps two feet (60 cm) or less. Thus, the enormous stress placed upon the delicate human visual system, for prolonged periods of time, requires constant focusing and precise eye teaming. Those all-important focusing muscles inside the eye tense up and become rigid. Relaxed viewing requires distances greater than those available in either a submarine, an office or in most schoolrooms. The longer our Yellow Submarine friends, office workers, and our schoolchildren remain in these visual prisons, the worse their vision problems may become.

Changes in vision were also noticed in Minutemen combat crew members who had been encapsulated, for certain periods, in small sealed chambers illuminated by sub-standard lighting. More specific eye measurements and additional testing revealed that, along with a decrease in vision, a definite increase in myopia (near-sightedness) was noticed in these men. This newly altered, visual situation was a reaction or adaptation to stress. Myopia is a vision problem which has profound physical, social, and psychological implications; it usually develops in a visually limited environment.

Picture yourself in the frozen wastes of the Arctic—hunting, fishing, shooting the rapids in a kayak, leading a life primarily devoted to survival in barren, hostile surroundings. Yet, there is no crowding-in of the environment, no artificial restrictions to impose any kind of stress upon vision. Myopia is virtually non-existent here.

When "civilization" came to Alaska it brought a new way of life to thousands of Eskimo children. What happened? The children no longer spent most of their time outdoors. Along with compulsory Western education, came beginners' reading groups and the visual stress of intense focusing and distance restriction, coupled with long hours of reading under inadequate light at home. Like our submariners, the young Eskimos were thrust into an unnatural, visual plight. Of all the children studied in Barrow, Alaska, 58 per cent, an exceptionally high percentage, showed signs of myopia. Over a period of time, the submarine sailors, the missile crews, and our Eskimo friends, all experienced the same biologically unacceptable near-point situation, which forces an individual to perform efficiently within a distance equal to the reach of his arm. Only through a change in visual behavior can the organism adjust to this situation.

Movement is the key to life; body movement the key to physical health, and eye movement the key to visual health. Sustained focusing in a restricted area of movement, within an unnatural environment produces stress. By visually shrinking the world and by giving up some measure of distance vision freedom, no longer needed for concentrated near-point activity—reading, writing, drawing—a person under stress is making it easier for himself to work close up.

Physiological optics, the science of vision, has shown that the near-sighted individual does not need to focus as much as others do for near-point activity. We believe it is this important focusing adaptation which actually causes environmentally induced myopia, whereby the visual system finds a way to reduce some of this imposed stress. The muscle that controls the focusing mechanism becomes cramped, spasmed, "charley-horsed," and can no longer relax for distance viewing. Distant objects become blurred and myopia sets in as a symptom of near-point stress.

We have just proposed an alternate way of looking at the development of myopia. The usually accepted reason for people becoming myopic is that it is a hereditary growth function. Many scientists have found this explanation to be inadequate. We actually believe that heredity may account for only a small percentage of myopia cases. Traditionalists in visual care cry that there are no means of remediation. The accepted method of treatment is to temporarily restore clear distance vision with glasses. According to our schema for the development of myopia, this would be tantamount to treating the symptoms of the problem, without finding its cause. In specific cases, if the symptoms are detected at the right time, we do have alternative means of treatment which are not new and have been known for many years.

Clinical evidence from private practitioners and results of visual research studies dealing with the effect of the environment's configuration on vision are available. Numerous studies have shown a significantly larger number of people who are involved with near-point activities suffering from myopia, compared to those engaged in less visually demanding occupations. Studies have been made of animals in captivity who became myopic; it is interesting that, statistically, less myopia has been found in country children compared to those living in cities. Improvement in vision following specialized training procedures, effectiveness of judicious lens application to stabilize myopia, flashes of clear vision in subjects under hypnosis, actual decrease in short-sightedness in children over the summer vacation, as well as numerous other examples, point to real possibilities for myopia control.

No longer should a negative lens that makes images seem smaller be prescribed to temporarily restore distance vision in every case. Such a lens forces a person to focus more and compounds the stress rather than alleviating it. The increased stress also seems to speed up the progression of myopia by frequently making it necessary for the individual to wear thick glasses which become thicker and thicker from year to year. A different type of lens, a positive "near lens" for near-centered work must be prescribed to relax the focusing muscles of the eye and relieve stress. This lens spreads the light that reaches the back of the eye over a larger area and in many cases seems to slow down progression of myopia. As this lens is placed before the eye of a person reading a book, it magnifies and causes an apparent movement or spatial shift of the book *away* from the reader. In this way, the lens creates an environmental condition more consistent with the natural functioning of the human visual system.

Before irreversible structural changes in the eye can occur, a correct lens, prescribed at the right time, and possibly supplemented by an individualized eye exercise program, can help distance vision to return to normal. In addition, this special "near lens" has been shown to bring about changes which are beneficial to the entire body, and not merely to the eyes, including improved posture, reduced back muscle tension, lower blood pressure, and a return to normal respiration and galvanic skin responses. This optimum lens also offsets other adverse bodily reactions and changes induced by stressful near-centered activity. Oscillations of the head and neck cease and visual performance becomes more efficient. Once this type of stress is alleviated, it has been found that patients are better prepared to achieve and to perform within the confines of their working environment.

D. B. Harmon, Ph.D., who specialized in the study of the processes of growth and development in the schoolchild, reported that a European ophthalmologist prophesied, as long as a century ago, that visual problems, principally myopia in schoolchildren, would result largely from bad lighting and adverse postural stresses induced by poorly designed school equipment. Dr. R. W. Lowry Jr., an optometrist* working with children, stated that as many as 70 per cent of all acquired vision problems originate from poor posture. This becomes meaningful when we hear that Duke Elder, M.D., found a significant portion of the visual fibers in man to be associated with lower primitive photostatic (light and posture) centers rather than with higher, sensory functions of vision.

---

*In England, an optometrist is known as an ophthalmic optician.

CHAPTER TWO

THE 20/20 MYTH

WHEN you go to have your eyes examined and can read the bottom line of an eye chart, you may be told that you have 20/20 vision and there is nothing wrong with your eyes. Millions of people all over the world are being led to believe that clear sight at distance automatically guarantees perfect vision. But 20/20 eyesight at distance is only one aspect of the entire realm of visual performance.

"Robert was completing third grade but was only able to read at first grade level. One year of special remedial help had resulted in frustration and little or no improvement. His mother brought him in for an optometric evaluation even though he had successfully scored '20/20' on a recent school distance vision screening test. The investigation revealed that he did indeed have 'perfect eyes' for distance seeing but was unable to team them up at the near reading distance. He saw double whenever he tried to read. In answer to his astonished mother's question why he had not

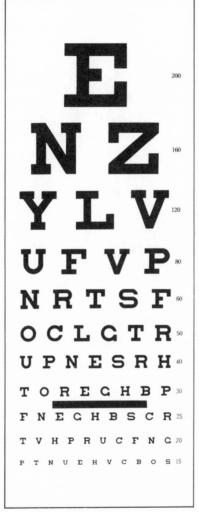

Courtesy: Bausch & Lomb

told her or his teacher of this before, he replied simply and honestly, 'I thought everyone saw that way!' "

(Adapted from R.C. Orem,
Learning to See, Seeing to Learn.)

The story of Robert and many like him shows that 20/20 vision does not necessarily assure visual efficiency at near-point reading, or even at far-point distance. Research studies reveal that a child that scores 20/20 sight can often be the poorer student—the under-achiever. This fact was borne out in a recent study by optometrist Dr. Arnold Sherman, relating vision disorders to learning disability. Out of a group of 50 children diagnosed by educators, psychologists and reading teachers as "learning disabled," Dr. Sherman found that although 45 had 20/20 vision, 46 were unable to use both eyes together as a team. Furthermore, a high percentage of mechanical and perceptual vision problems, unrelated to 20/20 distance vision, were found.

When primitive man stalked the grassy plains of this earth ten thousand years ago, he *had* to see from a distance to hunt and kill game for his food and clothing and to protect himself against predatory attacks. The ability to see far was a key factor in his survival. Ten thousand years ago, sharp and keen 20/20 vision was indeed an important physical asset. Many of today's traditional eye examinations, which often confirm the presence of 20/20 vision, would therefore have been adequate for the caveman and his life needs. BUT, SUCH TESTS ARE NOT FOR YOU!

Most of our important social and cultural demands are now placed within "arm's reach"—visually speaking. It is here that you must succeed. If you cannot master the printed word you will be lost. Emphasis has shifted from far to near, from the unrestricted to the restricted visual field, from open to confined space, from detection at distance to interpretation at arm's length. The fight for survival has shifted from the endless vistas of early man to the confined spaces in private homes and in educational institutions of modern man, and ultimately to the printed page.

Consequently, the end point of the traditional eye examination can only be the beginning of a complete vision analysis. It therefore becomes imperative to further investigate our *near visual world* and consider how it may even influence and modify our distance vision. Prescribing glasses on the basis of traditional *optical* theories to "correct" visual acuity problems completely neglects the *perceptual* aspects of vision, rendering the "dogma of 20/20" shortsighted in itself.

To communicate with the world around you, it therefore appears logical to consider not only a lens acceptable at far distance but also a lens which will provide the most efficient and the optimum visual performance within arm's reach—where you read the daily news, do your clerical work, ply your arts and crafts, or gaze into your lover's eyes.

CHAPTER THREE

FIX, FOCUS, AND FUSE

WE now know there is more to vision than 20/20 sight. It also includes fixation, the ability to direct our eyes accurately to what we are looking at to gather information. It is present soon after birth and the eye must develop through continued and constant use to improve this basic visual skill.

FIXATION

Question: "Doctor, I have noticed that my daughter moves her head as she reads. Her teacher tells me that she also moves her finger along the page while she reads. Does this have anything to do with eye movements?"

Answer: "Yes, these are examples of inefficient fixation and eye tracking. Your daughter's fixation ability is not sufficiently developed to divorce her body movements from her eye movements. She needs the support of her head and the guidance of her finger to help keep her place while she reads. The teacher who prohibits the use of this much needed support may be doing her more harm than good!"

A child's ability to move both eyes in the direction of the visual "target", to "lock-in" visually on this target and to promptly give up fixation of one object to reach for something else visually, is all part of the act which forms the foundation for *pursuits* and *saccades*, the more complex eye movement skills. While pursuits represent the ability to follow targets in motion smoothly and accurately, saccades represent the ability to move the eyes from one point to another in a jump-like fashion.

In his book, *The Slow Learner in the Classroom*, Newell C. Kephart, a psychologist, asks us to consider how difficult it would be for a child to read a passage if, when presented with the sentence "the mouse ran up the clock," the visual fixations involved were random. The child might then see—"the m he clo se ra p the . . . ", etc.

There seems to be a link between eye movements and emotions. We have observed that people who feel insecure often tend to avoid eye contact (direct fixation) with others during conversation. The question arises whether poor fixation is visual or emotional. We believe it could be both. If it is primarily a visual problem, relief of "fixation pain" through visual training would solve it. If, however, poor fixation arises from emotional problems, why not use visual training in psychological therapy? As research has revealed that pursuit ability in schizophrenic patients is generally poor, we are led to believe that a link does exist between eye movements and psychological instability.

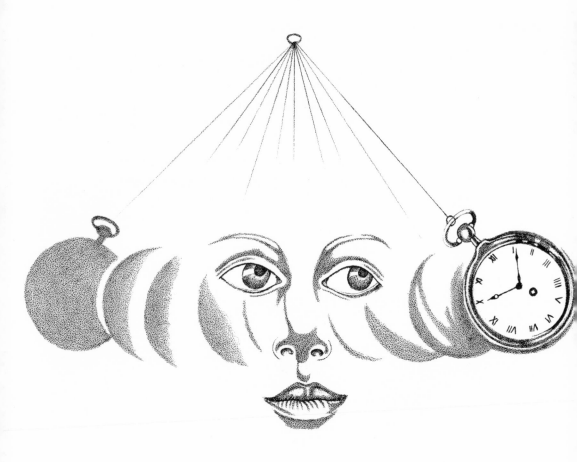

Fixational movements (pursuits) of the eye are needed to follow the swing of the watch on a string. Eye pursuits should be as smooth and as even as the path of a pendulum.

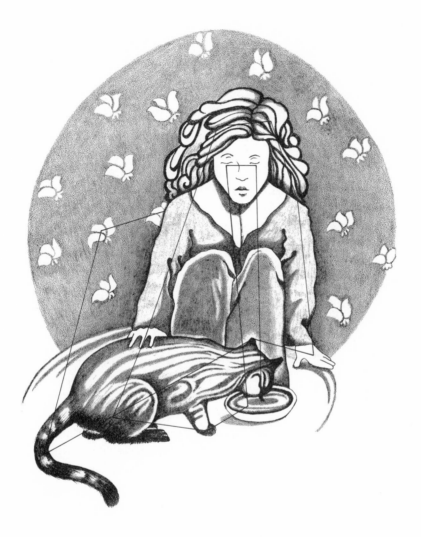

Jump-like movements (saccades) piece together and build up a concept or object of interest in the environment. The point-to-point lines indicate how a scene is being constructed and analyzed visually by saccadic eye movements.

FOCUS

We have often been asked whether it is true that the lens of a camera and the lens of an eye work in the same way. A glance at any old biology textbook will illustrate how strikingly similar the camera and the eye *seem* to be. It is not that simple, however. By moving a lens forward and backward to focus the image on film, the camera example makes vision appear as a passive, mechanistic process.

When your child shifts his gaze from distance to near, he must *accommodate* or focus his eye lens. Internal eye muscles control this important function. Each place he looks at requires a different focusing effort. The closer he looks, the more he has to focus. This is a dynamic process which constantly adjusts, seeks, and manipulates. If your child cannot focus well, especially after the strain of prolonged reading, he will experience foggy or blurred print, and his eyes will have to work harder to "make it clear."

A child who has trouble focusing is like a novice golfer who worries about his swing. While he concentrates on the mechanics of the swing, he is not paying full attention to actually striking the ball. The child, forced to concentrate on the mechanics of focusing, cannot pay full attention to his reading. As a result, concentration lags and he will tire after a short time. He is *wasting* energy and must de-focus, let go, to avoid pain.

Try this experiment:

Wear your distance glasses and close one eye. Look at the letter E on the following page. Pick up this book and slowly bring it closer and closer to your face, keeping the image of the E clear. Check one eye at a time. The letter E will soon go out of focus.

E

The ability to focus varies, depending on the age of different individuals. A child of ten can be expected to bring the letter to about 3 inches ($7\frac{1}{2}$ cm) from his face, before it goes out of focus, whereas for an adult, whose focusing ability decreases with age, the E would go out of focus at twice or three times that distance. Refer to the following Table of Expecteds to check how well a person of your age should do in this test.

TABLE OF EXPECTEDS

Age (Years)	Biological Variation of Focusing Distance of Letter E With Age:	
	Distance from Eyes	
10	.2.8"	7.1 cm
15	.3.3"	8.3 cm
20	.4.0"	10.1 cm
25	.4.7"	11.9 cm
30	.5.7"	14.4 cm
35	.7.2"	18.2 cm
40	.8.8"	22.3 cm
45	.11.4"	28.9 cm

The ability to focus properly and sustain this effort over a period of time will determine whether you carry over your distance acuity into the near world. It is crucial that you realize that 20/20 visual acuity at distance does not guarantee this ability.

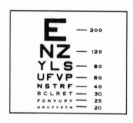

REDUCED SNELLEN CHART
Test distance: 16 inches (40 cm)

To check your near vision, one eye at a time, cup or cover one eye lightly without applying pressure, and hold this book 16 inches (40 cm) from your face. Wear your distance glasses. If you can read the bottom line of the Snellen Chart, you have successfully carried over 20/20 distance vision into your near world. If you cannot read the 20/20 line, but can read the line above it, you have only 20/25 vision in that eye; if you can only read the line above that, you have 20/30 vision, and so on.

With the following chart you can check a small child's near vision — one eye at a time. Because of the problem of communicating with preschoolers, start with the large pictures. Make sure you understand the child's word for the figures, whether he calls the bird a chicken, or the jeep a car. It is not necessary to correct him, just ensure that he is consistent throughout.

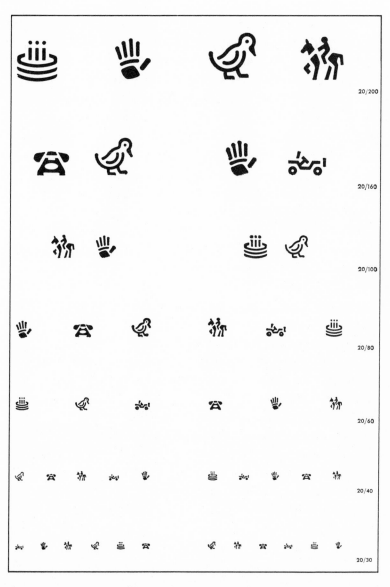

CHILD'S RECOGNITION AND NEAR POINT TEST CHART
Test distance: 13 inches (32'5 cm)

Courtesy: American Optical Corporation

Today, optometrists conduct various near point tests. Some of these tests do not even require you to answer questions. They help the optometrist to evaluate not only how well you can focus but also how well you can utilize the information gained from focusing. Do you understand what you see? Can you act upon this abstract information?

All these cognitive processes are intricately linked with focusing and represent a higher mental function. Scientists have proved that the focusing lens inside the eye constantly undergoes tiny oscillations, which represent a seeking and searching "what is it?"–"what am I looking at?" It is as if the lens focuses while the brain thinks.

We have been asked why ophthalmologists sometimes put drops in patients' eyes during examinations. These drops cut off the ability to focus, especially close up, for several hours.

The purpose of drops, known as mydriatics, is usually to dilate the pupils and thereby facilitate the internal examination of the eye. To better measure distance vision, however, a special drug known as a cycloplegic, which temporarily paralyzes the focusing mechanism, is sometimes used. For diagnostic purposes, the ophthalmologist does not want the focusing muscles to interfere with his distance measurements. Some eye specialists, however, neglect this focusing function; it should therefore be stressed that near vision cannot be evaluated effectively under such artificial conditions. The ophthalmologist may also use a cycloplegic to obtain additional comparative readings, following the regular, and sometimes difficult examination of children, or of children

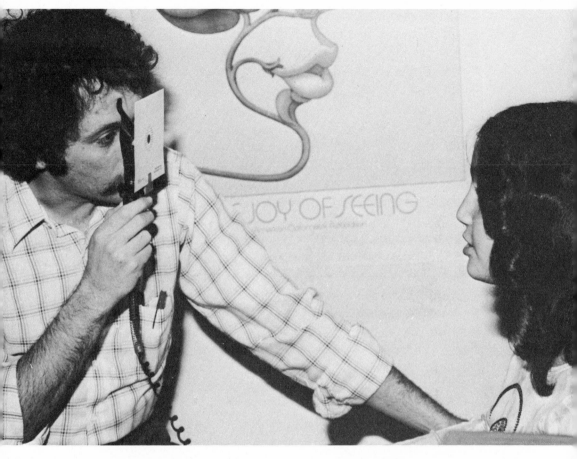

One of the objective tests used to evaluate visual competence at near point. The patient is asked to read the card while the doctor sights through the hole in the card.

whose responses are poor, those with variable focusing patterns, and crossed eyes cases.

Far-sighted children must sustain constant focusing efforts to keep vision clear while looking at a distance. How hard they have to work to maintain clear distance vision depends upon how far-sighted they are. Glasses are not only used for clear vision but also to help the child relax the focusing mechanism; they will also relieve fatigue and reduce tension and discomfort which result from excess energy expenditure.

Since 20/20 vision is not usually a factor with far-sighted children, the typical school screening test seems useless, as their far-sightedness frequently goes undetected in many routine examinations. An informed and alert teacher, a parent, or a school nurse can easily discover this type of problem. What are some of the signals that should make a parent suspect far-sightedness?

If your child complains of headaches in the forehead region or of nausea;

if you notice irritability or nervousness after prolonged reading;

if your child holds a book far away from his/her eyes;

if you detect poor attention span or general restlessness.

If other organic problems have been ruled out by your physician, your child may be far-sighted. Remembering that the closer we look the more we have to focus, it becomes obvious that the far-sighted child's real problem lies in dealing with near work;

there may be attempts to actually *avoid* close activities. The child might not like to sit and work with crayons and coloring books, cut-outs or building blocks, erector sets or bead threading. In fact, he might shy away from anything that involves near visual concentration. A far-sighted child may even conveniently lose books or misplace assignments, because he cannot compete with classmates, and wishes to escape embarrassment.

FUSION

We have *evolved* into two-eyed beings. Unlike Cyclops in Homer's *Odyssey*, we possess the ability to visually locate objects in the third dimension, assuming we have single, binocular vision.

This appreciation of depth, or stereopsis, represents the zenith of two-eyed vision; one-eyed Cyclops had none of this; he saw only straight ahead and on one plane. Being monocular he needed and probably used different clues to obtain a crude idea of where objects were in space.

Motion parallax, or the relative movement of near and far objects, was one clue. If you have ever looked at a distant object out of a train window, you might have noticed that while it seemed to take a long time to pass that distant object, another, closer object seemed to whiz by. It was this kind of concept that gave Cyclops a rough idea of how far away his supper was! Another clue was probably the result of his efforts to focus the lens in his one and only eye. To see his prey on the far horizon, he didn't need great focusing ability; yet, while devouring his kill, he had to focus harder, to see and savor what he was eating.

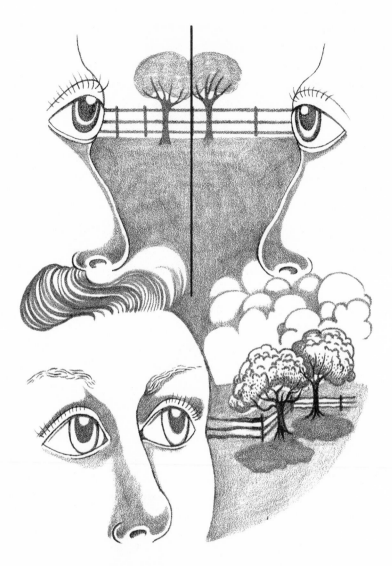

Two eyes have we,
Two different views,
Much advantage, many clues.
Two eyes, two pictures, here to see,
One plus one really equals three!

Just as a musical composition represents something more than a sequence of musical notes, so fusion represents something more than the simple summation of two ocular images. It provides a third dimension of sight. This quality gives us not only the ability to perceive the subtleties of space but also offers us the chance to extend our awareness.

To determine whether or not your eyes can bring about fusion, try the following simple test reproduced in color on the inside jacket of this book:

Hold a pencil close to the page with the lead centered between the two colored circles. Look intently at the tip of the lead; observe the circles on either side without looking directly at them. Slowly move the pencil towards your nose, always looking at the lead and keeping it, centered, until you see more than two circles; you might even see three or four.

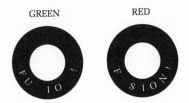

If you see three circles like this,

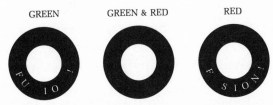

Courtesy: Keystone View Division of Mast/Keystone Company

stop moving your pencil. You have obtained fusion!

Note that the central fused circle is a "mixture" of the original red and green circles which will appear shiny and lustrous. The central, fused circle should contain the complete word FUSION. This central circle may appear to have an extra dimension of sight.

If you see *four* circles, don't be alarmed; this is the normal, physiological sign of two-eyed vision. Continue moving your pencil until you see the inner two circles approach each other and fuse. If you have undue difficulty performing this test, you may have a visual problem.

When you view a distant object, your eyes look straight ahead. When you shift your gaze to a near object, you must turn your eyes towards your nose. This movement of the eyes from forward, distant viewing to forward, near-point viewing is known as *convergence.*

Try this convergence test on your child: pick up a pencil and ask him to look at the tip. Bring it slowly towards his nose. You will see what your optometrist sees when he tests for convergence. Observe your child's eyes; if he cannot perform this act efficiently, one of his eyes will soon drift, usually outward, and he may complain of double vision. In this case, your child has limited convergence ability. If his skill is properly developed, he should be able to turn his eyes inwards when looking at an object, up to about 3 inches (7½ cm) from his nose. Faulty convergence produces rivalry between the two eyes and the resulting stress will bring about a drop in performance. Now ask someone to do this same test for you.

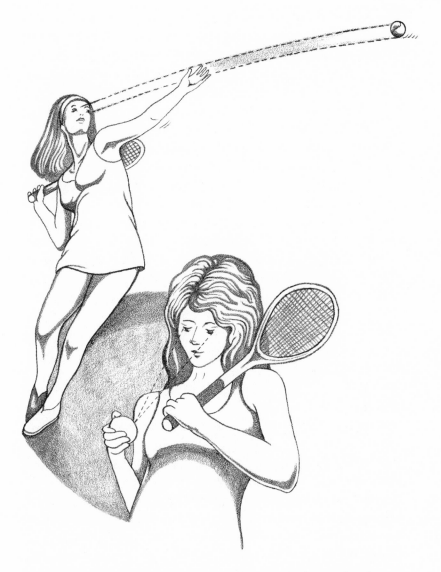

As she looks at the ball coming towards her the lines of sight are parallel.
The lines of sight triangulate on the ball, indicating convergence.

Many important seeing acts require both eyes to work well as a team. This is often overlooked in vision tests since eyes are frequently examined independently of each other and not as a team. Like focusing, this skill must be learned, guided, and developed. Whereas focusing attempts to answer the perceptual question "what is it?" eye teaming tries to answer "where is it?" Both these visual acts ultimately represent a higher mental function.

Does your child know exactly where objects are in relation to *where he is in space*? Jean Piaget, the eminent psychologist, believed that the development of a child's spatial world was of tremendous significance in overall perceptual development. Just as radar can determine the distance of objects away from the station, their direction, and their relationship to other things in space, a child's convergence system can essentially do the same. When the eyes converge, a visual triangle is set up with the object at the top and both eyes at the base.

This triangulating process tells the child where an object is located. Therefore, the candle on the table is seen to be in a certain direction and at a certain distance away from him. Adjacent objects automatically assume a spatial relationship to the candle and to the child, even though he is visually not directly tuned in on them. All objects and his interaction with them become more meaningful to him as he obtains an image of his environment and learns to "visually" feel and deal with it. He builds his own space world.

Picture a child tottering down a flight of stairs. He reaches for the banister and is confronted by two rails instead of one! A critical choice now faces him:

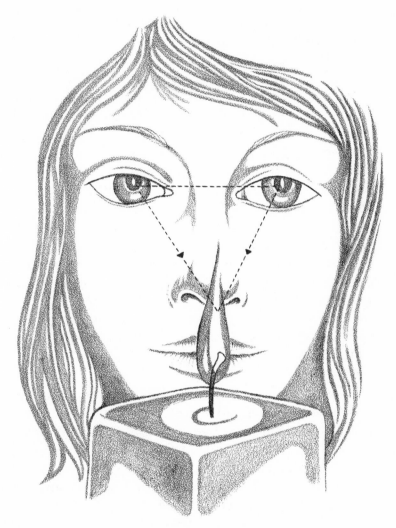

A visual triangle

which rail should he grab? To maintain clear, single vision eye teaming must be closely linked to focusing. To develop a flexibility between these two skills takes many years of practice.

Misalignment of the eyes can cause double vision. How can you detect double vision in your child? Look at his eyes; is one of them turned in or out, or up or down, in relationship to the other? Although it is not easy for an untrained observer to detect these conditions, except in cases of gross deviation, there are some *behavioral* indicators you can look for. Does your child tend to close one eye? Does he frequently rub one eye? Does he bump into things excessively? Does he elevate his chin and turn his head to one side using his nose to block out one half of his visual field? To avoid the confusion of double vision he might adopt all or some of these mechanical means to suppress or "turn off" vision in one eye.

The following is a test to determine whether you are suppressing vision in one eye, while you read. Are you using both eyes simultaneously?

Hold this book at a distance of about 16 inches (40 cm). Interpose a pen (or pencil) on your midline, halfway between your eyes and the text. Keep both eyes open and read the material. The pen should appear transparent and you should be able to read all the words on the page. None of them should be blocked out by the pen. Do not be concerned when two pens appear, as this is a normal, physiological phenomenon of two-eyed vision. If the pen does block out words and you must move your head to see around it, you are suppressing vision in one eye.

Seeing only one pen while you read is another sign that you are not using both eyes simultaneously. If you suspect the presence of double vision or other visual problems, seek professional help for yourself or your child; do not make your own diagnosis.

We have presented various visual skills and abilities and their individual significance in the total panorama of vision. It is meaningless to isolate one single skill from all the others, nor is it possible to obtain a complete visual-behavioral profile without a thorough analysis of the very complex act of vision and all its components.

CHAPTER FOUR

ENCOUNTERS WITH COMMERCIAL EYE CARE

WHILE working as a doctor in several commercial optical chains in New York City, I gained insight into the theories and practices of big business eye care. These chains are basically frame dispensing outlets with eye doctors usually practicing on the premises in order to increase the volume of sales. Eye doctors mean eye tests and eye tests mean prescriptions! New York is not the only city where such stores exist and do a thriving business!

What went on in some of these "shoptical" establishments served to convince me of the inferior standards of eye care they maintained. I was frequently criticized by the sales personnel for taking too long with my examinations and was told, in no uncertain terms, not to spend so much time with the "customers." Note that the people who came to have their eyes examined were called customers instead of patients. It was the sales staff who told the doctor how to do an eye examination, what type to give, and how long to take over it.

One day I was confronted by the store manager, an optician, trained and skilled in the making and dispensing of eye glasses. He questioned my methods of examination and warned me that I could not do "that sort of thing here." It seemed that by spending more time with a patient, I was upsetting his almost military type of operation. Apparently, optical managers such as he, usually receive a percentage of the company's profits. Of course, the more patients I saw, the more money he was likely to make.

At one establishment appointments were usually scheduled every fifteen minutes. I did not think that was long enough to examine a patient properly. However, I was surprised to find that even some of the patients got annoyed when they had to wait past their appointment time. They were upset because I took longer than the fifteen minutes they considered adequate for the type of eye test they had been used to receiving. What they had been getting and what they expected to get was a quick analysis of their visual needs. They had never undergone a thorough vision examination, and when they did allow me to test their eyes properly, the most frequent comment was, "Dr. Shapiro, none of the other doctors here have ever spent so much time with me; I never had an examination like this before!" The system under which these shops function cannot profitably operate and provide good patient care which leads to the kind of gratification I felt after comments such as these. Being merely profit-oriented, these establishments cannot possibly pay attention to the individual's visual "bill of rights."

During my time as a "shoptical" eye doctor, I worked in one department which had two examining units. My job was to act as the "back-up man" for the other doctor to lessen his load and to allow him to see at least one hundred and twenty patients in one single working day. To perform a competent vision analysis on one hundred and twenty patients would take a responsible practitioner at least two weeks!

In one place, the manager took it flagrantly upon himself to "examine" patients himself, although he was not a qualified optometrist. He told me it was quite easy, "All you do is measure their old glasses, fiddle around with the testing lenses until you think you are pretty close to the correct prescription, and bingo, the glasses can be ready in no time at all!" He admitted to me he had a little trouble fitting those people who had never worn glasses before.

The most tragic victims of such commercialized operations are inevitably children, as their visual systems are still developing. One day, after examining a little boy, I told his mother that he did not require glasses. She thanked me and after they had left the store, the optician-manager stared at the record card in disbelief and asked me why I had not prescribed glasses for the boy. "He does not need them," I said. "Well, you could at least have given him a pair with a tint for reading or something," he replied.

A study supervised by Dr. S. Friendly, of the Ophthalmology Department of the Children's Hospital National Medical Center in Washington, D.C., revealed that 72.4 per cent of children between the ages of 4 and 11 were "wearing glasses not corrected appropriately or adequately." In fact, 40 per cent of these children would have been better off without glasses!

A few years ago, following an investigation of "eyeglass emporiums" in New Jersey, the residents of the State were alarmed to read in their newspapers that at least one hundred of these establishments were giving "quickie" eye examinations lasting two to three minutes and were dispensing inadequate prescriptions. The investigations also revealed that many of the examiners were either insufficiently trained professionals or, in some cases, poorly qualified non-professionals. Specifically, out of a total of 36 *physicians* involved, only three had specialized training in eye care; only 18 out of 85 prescriptions were found to be adequate for the investigators' visual needs and out of 71 pairs of glasses bought by the investigators, 62 of the prescriptions were improperly filled.

I have found that some of these "emporiums," employed clever psychological tactics to condition patients towards acceptance of a new pair of glasses. As a "special concession," they were allowed to select their frames before entering the examining room! By the same token, the eye doctor was not exempt from this type of conditioning, as it was his job to see to it that the patient did not leave empty-handed.

I shudder to think how many thousands of middle-aged and elderly people never undergo glaucoma checks when they visit their friendly neighborhood optician. After cataracts, this disease is the leading cause of blindness. Glaucoma is easily detected with a tonometer, an instrument which measures pressure in the eyeball. When I asked one manager why he did not have one on his premises, he told me he was afraid of lawsuits resulting from possible damage to the eye! What an absurd statement! I have used tonometers that do not even touch the eye.

The average person who frequents these "shoptical" establishments does not realize that the 20/20 test is the only eye service that can possibly be rendered effectively by their staff. Some of the optometrists who work in these places realize they are administering inferior care, "Schlock Care" as they themselves refer to it, but admit they do it for financial reasons. Other eye doctors are satisfied to practice in a very narrow sense, giving 20/20 tests and believing they are doing a good job. They are either not aware of or do not want to hear about the tremendous progress in modern eye care that has been made in recent years.

To arrive at a sound diagnosis, a complete eye examination should record the general medical history, the medical eye history, the complaints, and the environmental demands of a patient. You can never have too much information.

Before vision analysis can begin, a thorough investigation of possible presence of ocular disease should be made. A pathological work-up includes eye muscle evaluation and testing pupillary reflexes, and external as well as internal ocular tissue integrity. Anyone over the age of thirty-five, or anyone suspected of having increased eye pressure, must have a glaucoma test. Vision analysis must also include an evaluation of focusing and eye teaming skills, with testing done at distance and within arm's length.

You might have had a highly professional eye examination and received the best in visual care, but this becomes meaningless in the face of inferior optical work. Some establishments will give you cheap or warped lenses, lenses with imperfections, or off-centered lenses. They can get away with these practices if the patient does not complain of nausea, dizziness, or other discomfort.

Optometrists provide a complete eye care service and check their own lab work. Most ophthalmologists do not dispense their own prescriptions, and it therefore becomes imperative that you take your glasses back for verification. Remember, there's more to checking a prescription than just verifying lens centers and making sure the strength of the glasses is correct. If you are dissatisfied, even if your doctor maintains your prescription is correct, complain! It may be the shape of the lens, i.e. the base curve, which alters your perception and causes you discomfort. Such problems can be rectified.

When acquiring glasses, don't forget that proper fitting frames to suit your face are essential. Frames that do not fit may diminish the effectiveness of the prescription and may reduce a child's willingness to wear glasses.

Free eye tests, bargain specials and advertised one-hour service, all constitute the sucker's bait that lures the unwary into the store. Millions of people belonging to various unions—police, fire-fighters, teachers, teamsters, etc., and their families—each enjoying their own special discount rates, may be getting "wholesale" vision care; but is it adequate?

Commercial eye care is big business, not a profession. The doctor's office becomes a store and frequently a factory. The patient becomes a customer; the doctor ultimately a technician. The situation is perhaps best summed up by Dr. Milton J. Eger's editorial in the Journal of the American Optometric Association:

> "The unethical commercialist is the most detrimental of all. He is honest enough to admit to the world that he is selling glasses at a price and will stoop to anything to 'make a buck.' He places a price on everything, a value on nothing. Personal gain is his only goal . . . the patient be damned. He runs the gamut of every trick in the trade toward his objective. Every eye practitioner is his competitor: he has no colleagues. He walks the tightrope of the laws of his state and is constantly a thorn in the side of the profession. To him, optometry is not only a business, but one without ethics or morality. To him, this is a pure and simple economic fight for the eye care dollar with no holds barred."

Dubious optical practices are not restricted to the United States. In Canada, for instance, a unique situation exists. Consumer complaints that eyeglass prices were too high, and charges by certain independent optical companies that activities by two large manufacturers and distributors of ophthalmic appliances, materials, and equipment were making it difficult for them to operate, led to an investigation by the Federal Restrictive Trade Practices Commission. Nationwide hearings began early in 1976 to find out if price or quality of glasses and accessories were affected by the domination of the market by these companies. If the allegations brought out during these hearings are found to be factual, it is hoped the Canadian federal government will recommend to the provincial governments who are responsible for the administration of health care, that legislation be introduced, limiting the monopolistic control of the optical industry.

A ban on advertising ophthalmic products exists in all Canadian provinces except Ontario, British Columbia and Manitoba. George Adamson, general manager of King Optical Company, would like to see this ban removed in the other provinces. He maintains, the assumption that price advertising in the field contributes to a lowering of quality is not necessarily true.

He would also like to see the major optical manufacturers and distributors divest themselves of enormous financial interests in the retail field, and believes their outlets should operate under their own names to make consumers aware who they are buying from, and to provide more genuine competition. After World War II, the same situation existed in the United States. Threatened with anti-trust legislation, the large optical companies voluntarily divested themselves of their retail outlets to avoid government prosecution.

It must, however, be said in defence of one major manufacturer, Imperial Optical in this case, that they have brought eye care to countless remote communities, some as far north as the Yukon Territory, as well as to smaller towns in Eastern and Western Canada. Because of their vast financial resources, they were able to set up outlets in places where independent opticians could not have found a large enough clientele to operate profitably.

As an example of how to counteract the ever-present conflict of interest which still exists elsewhere in the eye care field, the Ontario government ruled in 1975 that members of the College of Optometry must not "rent or use any premises from a vendor of ophthalmic appliances, materials and equipment" nor "engage in the practice of optometry where any of the public entrances or exits of an optometrist's premises are within the premises of a retail merchant, optical company or ophthalmic dispenser." Optometrists and opticians have until 1979 to divorce their operations, and function independently. The authorities have also ruled that it is illegal for an optometrist to "own, or financially benefit from the operation of a company, firm or business that manufacturers, fabricates, supplies or dispenses ophthalmic appliances."

It can, therefore, be considered a step in the right direction that opticians in Ontario can no longer employ optometrists on staff. However, it is legal in Ontario for a person to engage in the practice of optometry with a qualified medical practitioner, logically an ophthalmologist.

Optometrists and ophthalmologists, especially recent graduates, allegedly received credit and loans from Imperial Optical. William Omand, a former employee with the company during the early seventies testified under oath during the Restrictive Trade Practices Commission hearings that he was involved with reviewing and discussing with senior management accounts receivable records for such financing. "There were underlying reasons in most cases as to whether interest would be charged or payment demanded....", he said. Some ophthalmologists were considered "important" to the company "because of the number of prescriptions that come from them through Imperial subsidiary retail dispensing locations."

When Mr. Omand was asked whether, while he was with the company, he knew of any system for monitoring the monthly performances by ophthalmologists and optometrists in terms of where the prescriptions went or how many were received by Imperial outlets, he confirmed that this type of system existed. The company has denied any wrongdoing.

The results of these hearings are to be published shortly.

CHAPTER FIVE

THE SPECIALIST'S VERDICT

WHILE working with New York ophthalmologists, all excellent surgeons and experts in their field, several incidents occurred which prompted me to examine the fundamental differences in approach to visual problems which exist within the ophthalmic profession. I was appalled to find that many top eye specialists who practice according to traditional methods are not reluctant to advise patients with common problems to accept their "visual fate" without question.

By citing three case histories, I hope to demonstrate why I do not agree with the finality of diagnostic verdicts brought in by some eminent men.

THE SHORT-SIGHTED EYE DOCTOR

Allan, a young schoolboy of about 14, came to see me one day, complaining of blurred distance vision which, he noticed, had become progressively worse over the last year or so.

Due to increased schoolwork, he had been doing a great deal of reading. "When I look up after long periods of reading, everything out there is foggy, Dr. Cohen!" he exclaimed. I gave him a complete visual analysis and discovered that his distance vision was a little below normal, less than 20/20, although he could see quite well up close. This was a typical case of myopia (short-sightedness), as taught and understood by many practicing eye doctors today.

I also discovered a focusing problem; Allan seemed unable to relax his focusing mechanism properly. This resulted in blurred distance vision whenever he looked up. Furthermore, there was a tendency for his eyes to turn further inwards than they should have done, a sign of poor eye teaming and stress. These two findings often go hand in hand in cases of beginning short-sightedness.

Based on these and other observations, plus the fact he had never worn glasses before, I decided to give him a dual-focus (bifocal) lens. The top of the lens would be plain window glass and the bottom part, prescription-ground to relax his focusing and allow for better eye teaming. I also hoped this lens would help prevent further deterioration in his distance vision.

"This lens is basically for school- and homework," I told Allan, "especially for prolonged reading periods."

To receive the best of care, a second medical opinion is important. The ophthalmologist who worked with me saw Allan, and later confronted me with my prescription, "I really think you're wrong," he said. "He's too young for bifocals, they're expensive, look ugly, and I don't see how this will help him!" I explained my rationale for the prescription. "Don't you see," he continued, "it's just the normal course of his disease; he could become short-sighted at any age, and I don't think excessive reading has anything to do with it. I shall give him a pair of glasses to correct his blurred distance vision. If he wears them all the time, it will make him see like a normal person."

"Why should he have to wear glasses all the time if he can see quite well without them for close work? He'll only become more dependent on them," I interjected. "What about when he takes them off, does he see normally then?" But my colleague could not be persuaded ...

Two different ways of looking at visual problems result in two different ways of treating them. Can both be correct?

QUANTITY VERSUS QUALITY

One day I examined a girl of about 10 years of age. She was far-sighted. On testing her near vision I discovered she could not read the 20/20 line with either eye. Just then the ophthalmologist with whom I worked, came into the room.

"This is interesting," I said, "she cannot read the bottom line of our near-vision chart; she could have a focusing problem." "Nonsense!" he replied, "she is too young for that and should have plenty of reserve focusing power to overcome her far-sightedness; she should have no problem reading the chart." Of course, as a young girl she would have a high potential focusing power. According to our Table of Expecteds (page 25), a 10-year-old can focus a small letter E as close as 2.8 inches (7 cm) from the face.

The ophthalmologist suggested we dilate her

eyes and check for possible disease. No evidence of disease could be found. Try as I might, I could not convince him that she might have a problem utilizing her high focusing potential. It is not only the *degree* of far- or near-sightedness that causes visual symptoms to emerge, but the small errors, subtle anomalies, and the *quality* of response that can be just as devastating to visual functioning as any large and obvious deviations.

As the ophthalmologist was more concerned with the gross quantity of the girl's focusing power rather than with its quality, she walked out of the office with the same problem with which she had come in.

PRAY FOR VISION!

An interesting incident occurred during a confrontation with another ophthalmologist over treatment of a "lazy eye." This condition is one of reduced vision which cannot be improved to 20/20 status with lenses alone (Amblyopia).

James was a second-year architectural student, 21 years old. He was on his way to a summer semester in France and had come to see us for a check-up before leaving.

I did a preliminary work-up and a refraction (vision test). James wore thick glasses and was extremely short-sighted, so much so that I concluded that he must have been born this way, as this type of short-sightedness is rare. His left eye had fairly good vision, around 20/30, but try as I might, I could not improve his right eye to beyond 20/400 which is very poor indeed.

On further testing I discovered that his right eye tended to drift outward from time to time, a phenomenon that occasionally accompanies poor vision in one eye.

James was aware of his condition and asked me whether anything could be done about it. "Quite possibly," I replied. "If there is no disease process at the back of your eye, in other words, if your eye is healthy, we might be able to improve your vision by patching your good left eye and forcing your right eye to work more. Some eye exercises would probably speed up this process. Once vision in your right eye has improved, we could work on coordinating both eyes and teach you how to use them together. Although you are already 21, I believe we can help you. However, you must realize that it could take longer at your age than if you were five or six years old." James appeared willing to try.

The eye surgeon on staff saw him for a follow-up examination. This is what he told James: "Your eyes seem healthy. The problem of your right eye cannot be resolved. I do not think occlusion (patching) will work, as you are too old for it. Your right eye will probably drift even further out as you get older and eventually you might need surgery. In the meantime, the only thing you can do, is pray!"

One problem – two approaches. Who is the loser?

CHAPTER SIX

THE POLITICS OF EYE CARE

IDEALLY, Ophthalmology, Optometry, and Opticianry—the Three O's—should be separate professions; they should function separately. However, circumstances have created a redundancy of services with varying degrees of quality, and although each discipline is all-inclusive, it cannot function in isolation.

Around the world, the eye care field is plagued by politics and behind-the-scenes disputes, as the Three O's battle each other for professional supremacy in their "Three-Ring Circus."

THE THREE-RING CIRCUS

RINGMASTER: Ladies and Gentlemen! Welcome to our Three-Ring Circus! We have gone to extraordinary lengths, transcended many barriers, to bring to you those exponents of our profession who are willing to publicize their positions. Tonight, for your entertainment, we have gathered together, for the first time in the same arena, THE THREE O'S—

OPHTHALMOLOGY – OPTOMETRY – OPTICIANRY! Each will perform its own special act. Tonight you will hear from the experts, never-before-disclosed secrets, behind-the-scenes activities, and new revelations about eye care! Ladies and Gentlemen! In Ring No. 1, we proudly present: Ophthalmology!

OPHTHALMOLOGY: Ladies and Gentlemen! I have completed my medical training, including a three-year residency in my chosen specialty. I have been schooled in the skills of ocular surgery and the treatment of eye diseases. I prefer to operate and heal eyes, rather than waste my time testing vision. Anyone can test vision. I am the true eye specialist – I should have final say!

RINGMASTER: And now in Ring No. 2: Optometry!

OPTOMETRY: I have at least six years of specialized college education. I have been trained in eye anatomy, physiology, and pathology; neural anatomy and physiology; psychology of vision, including studies of physiological, geometrical, physical, and mechanical optics as well as in the clinical visual sciences. I specialize in vision for the partially-sighted, the application of contact lenses, pediatric vision, industrial and environmental vision, and vision training. I am the true vision specialist!

RINGMASTER: And now in Ring No. 3: Opticianry!

OPTICIANRY: I have two years' education in the theoretical and practical aspects of ophthalmic dispensing. I can measure, adapt, make, and deliver such devices as spectacles, contact lenses, artificial eyes, and low vision aids. Because of my skills to use measuring devices, instruments, machines, and hand tools, I serve the public in much the same manner as the pharmacist who fills your doctor's prescriptions. I am the specialist in ophthalmic dispensing!

RINGMASTER: The Three O's have introduced themselves. Let us set these three rings in motion so that you may watch our contestants in the "Battle for Your Eyes."

OPHTHALMOLOGY: You guys in Optometry! You call yourselves doctors, but can you really detect diseases? How many people are going blind because of undiagnosed glaucoma?

OPTOMETRY: We have extensive practical and academic training in the detection of eye diseases, including glaucoma. Today we use the same diagnostic instruments as you do. It's high time you visited some of our professional schools, attended our conventions, and read our journals. Come and see what we are doing; times have changed!

OPHTHALMOLOGY: It only takes a few months to learn how to test vision. You guys go to school for too long to learn your trade.

OPTOMETRY: There is a lot more to vision than clear sight. If you had studied more about it at your schools, you would better understand why we perform all those vision tests you call "sophisticated" and consider superfluous. Although you downplay vision, you spend most of your time measuring it and prescribing eyeglasses. Do what you have been trained to do!

OPTICIANRY: You guys in Optometry! You just want to sell glasses. Concentrate on examining eyes and leave the eyeglass dispensing to us!

OPTOMETRY: Only the unethical commercialist is out to push glasses. Most of us are concerned with quality eye care; eyeglass dispensing is secondary. It is you, the Opticians, who help perpetuate an evil system. On the other hand, you Ophthalmologists have turned to vision testing to supplement your incomes. We know there is not enough surgery and disease around to keep you busy. You no longer send us your prescriptions, for fear of losing patients. You are hiring opticians to work for you, right in your own offices.

OPHTHALMOLOGY: Some of our lens prescriptions do go to ethical and reliable optometrists; we do value their referrals. Besides, what right do you have to control the entire eyeglass market?

OPTOMETRY: Your appointment books are packed; patients must wait for months to see you. It is impossible to administer quality eye care and follow sound ophthalmological procedures while carrying such a heavy workload. How can you avoid cutting corners? Besides, you know that 93 per cent of people with eye problems actually have vision problems. Why not send them to us, the Vision Care Specialists?

OPHTHALMOLOGY: Too many people are going without eye care. It is our duty to examine everyone. We have even invented a machine—the Ophthalmetron—so that we can screen more and more patients. Just think, in three seconds we can get a 20/20!

OPTOMETRY: By trying to replace us with machines and technicians, you are setting the stage to exclude us from national health insurance schemes.

OPHTHALMOLOGY: Skilled technicians, that's all you are! Quit trying to be more than that.

OPTICIANRY: Yeah, that's all you are, technicians. All we need ophthalmologists and optometrists for, is to give us prescriptions.

OPTOMETRY: Doctors of Ophthalmology! You use your titles to wield power and attract patients who look to you as the specialists in eye care. Stop this cultural mystique of medicine! It distorts the true picture of eye care delivery.

RINGMASTER: Ladies and Gentlemen! May I interrupt? I have just been handed a ruling from the American Medical Association. It reads:

> "RESOLVED, that it is unethical for any doctor of medicine to teach in any school or college of optometry, or to lecture to any optometric organization, or in any way to impart technical, medical knowledge to non-medical practitioners."

Ladies and Gentlemen, you have seen the Spectacle of the Three O's. Does it make sense? Ah! Money–Money–Money! To bring order out of chaos, to promote organization within diversity, the Three O's must interlock constructively.

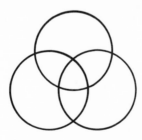

Optometrist Dr. Marjorie S. Ross, states; "Each discipline within the eye care field is, in fact, independent but interdependent in the total health care scheme. Though it is nearly impossible for any one discipline to prescribe the mode of practice of another, it would seem to be in the best interest of the public that all of us within the eye care field endeavour to provide the finest possible care at the least cost. This cannot be done when any one member of the eye care team functions at a level other than his training would determine ... "

As a patient, you are entitled to the best vision care possible. In seeking out this care, follow these useful guidelines:

- Anyone with red eye, eye infection, severe eye pain, sudden visual loss, or trauma to the eye, should immediately consult an ophthalmologist or visit an eye clinic at a hospital.
- Your child should receive a complete professional vision examination before entering kindergarten, ideally at age 3. Consult a competent optometrist.
- Throughout their teens, students should have annual check-ups, to insure early detection and possible prevention of vision problems.
- The American Optometric Association Committee recommends that all students in the lower third of the class, particularly those who possess the ability to achieve standards above their percentile rating, should be referred for complete vision analysis. Every student in the class, even those who are achieving but not working to within reasonable

limits of their capacity, should be referred for a complete optometric examination.

- Since demands on vision are relatively stable from age 20 to 35, we recommend an eye examination every two years during that period.
- Over 35, people should undergo eye examinations once a year. Presbyopia, a normal loss of focusing ability, then becomes a reality and chances of eye disease, such as glaucoma or cataracts, increase.
- Above 60, chances of eye disease are even greater. We recommend annual check-ups for this age group.
- Many optometrists who practice functional behavioral aspects of vision—the extended view—likely belong to the worldwide Optometric Extension Program, an organization which pioneered vision research and education.
- The College of Optometrists in Vision Development (C.O.V.D.) is an elite group of vision care specialists. A list of their members can be obtained by writing to C.O.V.D. Headquarters, P.O. Box 285, Chula Vista, California, 92012.
- To obtain a list of optometrists who practice vision training in the United States contact your local or state optometric society, or the Chairman of the Committee on Orthoptics and Vision Training, American Optometric Association, 7000 Chippawa Street, St. Louis, Missouri, 63119. In Canada, contact your provincial or federal optometrists' associations and the colleges of optometry at the University of Montreal in Quebec and at the University of Waterloo in Ontario.

- We feel sure your present eye doctor is competent to handle your visual needs.
- However, if anyone, anywhere in the world is in doubt as to where to obtain professional eye care, any professional, optometric and/or ophthalmological college or institution can be contacted for treatment.

CHAPTER SEVEN

STRESS
AND VISION
PROBLEMS

VISION problems are rampant in our complex society of today. The number of such problems in schoolchildren around the world is incredibly high and has passed epidemic proportions. A warning issued some time ago by the United States Public Health Service included the prediction that the number of American children under fifteen with vision problems would increase to seventy-five million by 1975.

In a way, the eyes of the preschool child can be likened to those of primitive man, as neither time nor environment have yet taken their toll. It is from Grade 2 onwards that biological, behavioral, and psychological visual stresses are first encountered. At this point, the child starts the complex process of reading to learn, not learning to read. Sitting for longer periods with restrained body movements requires tremendous visual and physical stamina. Greater mental effort is involved to comprehend and greater visual effort is required to focus in on words as the print becomes smaller and the space between the lines diminishes. Stronger fusion and more flexible focusing systems are necessary for reading to learn. These skills are the first to suffer under the shadow of prolonged stress.

Grade 1

I like to go to the zoo. I can see the animals in the zoo. I can see:
a lion
a tiger
an elephant.
Can you see the animals? What are they doing?
The lion is lying in the grass.
The tiger is walking up the hill.
The elephant is drinking water.

Joan and Maria became friends. After school, they walked home together. In the spring they played hopscotch in the park. In the winter, they went to the arena, and Joan taught Maria how to skate.

"Come to my house and have some hot chocolate," Joan said to Maria one day. "I am sorry, but I cannot come," replied Maria. "Why not," said Joan, "we could have so much fun, and I could show you my dolls and our little poodle." But Maria shook her head, and walked away.....

People are different, yet every person has certain basic needs. Some are physical while others are mental, emotional and social.

Your basic physical needs include shelter, protection from cold and heat, and enough food and sleep to give you energy, and keep you physically fit. To stay healthy you also need exercise, fresh air, and sunshine.

For teenagers and adults to enjoy good mental health, certain personal needs must be met. For instance, everyone has a need to love and be loved; a need for independence, a need for approval, and the desire to belong and be part of a group. Your happiness, well-being, and feeling of security depend on whether or not your physical and personal needs were met since you were born.

In addition to cross-sectioned studies, new improved methodologies are required to provide some experimental basis for the existence of these hyper-sensitive phenomena.

We must stress the significance of this theory, in the light of recent research studies which will lead to infinitely more conclusive and conceptually superior solutions.

Let us, therefore, examine the procedure in more detail, by collecting data relevant to the theory under scrutiny.

According to Darell B. Harmon, Ph.D., who specialized in the study of growth and development in the schoolchild, with emphasis on interaction among mind, body, and visually-centered aspects of learning, the organic child has just so much energy to expend. This energy must go toward satisfying basic needs to stay alive; converting food into usable chemical forms; protecting the child against infection and other disease threats; growing; and furnishing the energy for all the activities and adjustments the environment demands. Only a limited amount of energy is really free for activity. When these environmental demands exceed the energy free and available for this purpose, the child is deprived of some other vital needs and growth suffers first in most cases. Continued stresses are produced by poorly designed furniture, poor distribution of light, or poor visual performance. These environmental demands, inconsistent with basic performance patterns, might readily use up energy required for body growth, for protection against infection, or to overcome other adverse factors in a child's total surroundings. Harmon further stated that "as the child continues to grow in such surroundings, the final results are assymetrical or unbalanced body structures, deviating performances or physical and psychological lesions and disabilities."

Whenever environmental demands exceed the individual's visual tolerance over a period of time, visual deterioration sets in and adaptation begins. Look around and you will see how many of your adult friends wear glasses—outward signs of stress-induced vision adaptation. How many others do not wear glasses and walk around in a state of visual tension?

The concept of time and environmental impact are both considered in the behavioral approach to vision problems. Generally speaking, time plus adverse environmental demand equals stress-induced visual adaptation.

Adaptation is an attempt to make us as comfortable as possible within our environmental demands. Unfortunately, this attempt often results in a tradeoff, as it only allows us to function through a restricted range. The organism becomes warped while trying to maintain efficiency. As visual adaptation occurs, the individual may suffer a loss of distance vision resulting in myopia, or he may lose the ability to maintain two-eyed teaming resulting in a manifest eye turn.

Another type of adaptation to stressful visual tasks is purely academic; it is a breakdown in information processing which may result in, among other problems, poor reading comprehension. Individuals, with this type of adaptation pattern usually maintain intact visual systems (20/20 and straight eyes). They represent a portion of the so-called "learning disabled" or "dyslexic" population—children who are not achieving full potential. These types of adaptation are usually not clear-cut entities, but exist as varying combinations.

Other visual adaptations include high degrees of far-sightedness, astigmatism, amblyopia (lazy eye), and anisometropia (imbalances in the visual patterns between the two eyes). Often, the end result of such adaptations is the development of postural warps (head tilts, shoulder slumps, curved spines, etc.).

Contemporary men and women, confronted daily by stresses in their environment, are undoubtedly visually at risk. Pushed beyond physiological limits at school and at work, unable to cope with increasingly higher workloads, they seek escape. How can they minimize stress? How do they escape? Apart from adaptation, they have two alternatives:

Retreat from the Task or Job:

The White House Conference on Juvenile Delinquency and other studies have verified that "up to 80 per cent of delinquents had learning difficulties, specifically in reading ... and poor vision was found to be a contributing factor in 50 per cent of these cases. The involvement of young people in crime is especially tragic when many of them might have progressed in a normal manner if they had been provided with adequate visual care."

Continue the Task under Duress:

Maintain achievement at any cost. Result: mysterious symptoms or complaints.

Whichever route modern men and women take depends upon an individual's personality and his or her physical stress tolerances, as well as on various social pressures he or she may be subjected to at home, at school, and at work.

Stress-induced vision adaptations are not fixed. Just because the eyes and the body have adjusted to the situation does not mean the adaptation is irreversible. Many vision problems are trainable as we are able to alleviate most of their symptoms through judicious lens application, exercises and visual hygiene rules. This is a far cry from the traditional viewpoint that vision problems are innate, predetermined, and permanent. Yet, they tend to have a sinister quality about them; they appear, often disguised in different ways and may not become obvious until their manifest signs (myopia, eye turns, head tilts, lazy eye, etc.) surface. It is unlikely that anyone would even think of seeking professional help before that time.

CHAPTER EIGHT

IF WE
ONLY HAD
ONE EYE

THERE may be more to two-eyed problems than "meets the eye." They can be diverse and obscure and seem far removed from our visual system. As a result, they are often misdiagnosed and naturally mistreated, especially when symptoms from physiological causes parallel those from psychological causes.

The following three case histories reveal some of these problems.

THE NEUROTIC WHIPLASH VICTIM

One day in October, Miss F.G. was driving home after work. She went through an intersection and was suddenly forced to stop for another car. Applying her brakes, she heard a sickening thud from behind. The collision snapped her head back, and sent a sharp pain soaring through her lower back. . . .

So begins a most unusual and puzzling case of whiplash injury; a case so misleading and confusing in its complexity of symptoms that it baffled half a dozen medical specialists.

A whiplash injury, in its simplest terms, is the result of a violent flexion (bending) and extension (straightening) of the head and neck following the impact of two automobiles; it is a fairly common aftermath of rear-end collisions. When subsequent medical investigation and X-rays show no signs of structural damage, the injury should respond well to treatment and disappear altogether if given enough time.

For months after the accident, Miss F.G. suffered severe head, neck, and back pains. She was seen by an internist, an orthopedic surgeon, two ophthalmologists, and a neurologist. After extensive physiotherapy, traction, and pharmaco-therapy failed to give relief to headaches and other complaints, she was hospitalized and her back operated upon.

The neurologist's report revealed a bewildering array of symptoms: "She states that immediately before coming to hospital, her headaches were very severe. She could not sleep and blacked out for fifteen minutes. She was sick for an entire evening, but did not vomit. She has had momentary 'blackouts' since coming out of hospital. She gets a dizzy feeling at the top of her head. She staggers to the right. Her headache is worse on getting up. She had neck traction applied eight or nine days ago which helped some, but which did not completely relieve her headache. On closer questioning, she says she has occasionally vomited with the headaches; she has a ringing in her ears. Since the accident her arms have sometimes felt numb. She has trouble hanging on to things and has dropped instruments in her employer's office. She complains of twitching in her left arm on occasion, but not all the time. She states her back is much better since surgery. At times her vision is blurred and she has trouble focusing; this has happened three or four times since surgery. She has had trouble hearing and understanding what people say but has no real loss in hearing."

The neurologist's report concluded with the opinion that Miss F.G.'s headaches were due to "tension." He could find no organic or pathologic disorder. The ophthalmologist who examined her took an extensive case history and noted all her visual complaints: occasionally blurred vision, periodic double vision, difficulty in changing focus from distance to near and vice versa, sharp pains around her eyes. He concurred with the neurologist: "No eye findings, pathological or otherwise, to account for her complaint. She is a myope and her present correction is adequate." (She had 20/20 vision in both eyes.)

Because no pathological or functional problem related to the accident itself could be found, the consultants suggested her complaints were caused by an "anxiety tension state with hysterical overlays" and that psychiatric help be secured.

Six months after the accident, her physician made a startling discovery. He found that bandaging one eye for a day afforded her noticeable relief. Here was the first clue—evidence of a two-eyed problem! She was referred to Dr. Raymond R. Roy, an optometrist practicing in that area.

At the time, Miss F.G.'s pain was so intense that she had to be seen with her neck brace in place. A slight change in her glasses to compensate for an increase in myopia was temporarily prescribed while she went through a standard period of eye patching.

During that time, she noticed her head and neck tensions had considerably lessened. A few days later, Dr. Roy saw her again. This time, *definite clinical evidence of two-eyed stress was found.* Further intensive binocular testing resulted in the dispensing of a special temporary prismatic lens which compensated for Miss F.G.'s two-eyed imbalance. One week later, having worn these special prisms constantly, Miss F.G. reported her headaches were almost gone; she could be without her neck brace for several hours at a time and drive her car without feeling nauseous. The only remaining symptom was a mild dizziness.

Eventually, a new permanent prismatic lens was prescribed. By July, nine months after the start of her ordeal, Miss F.G. was "busy and active and leading a normal life." To all intents and purposes, she was completely cured.

A NON-ALCOHOLIC SOLUTION

Mr. F.F., a 32-year-old executive, had suffered from daily headaches for several years. They occurred in a most unusual pattern: starting at about 11 a.m., they disappeared during his lunch break and reappeared when Mr. F.F. resumed his afternoon activities. They were accompanied by intense nausea which continued as long as he was busy doing desk work. When he closed his eyes for brief periods, the pain was partially relieved.

Mr. F.F. concluded that the headaches must be associated with his eyes and consequently sought ophthalmological advice. He could not be helped. He consulted other medical specialists—a neurologist, a gastroenterologist, an internist, and a cardiologist.

An otolaryngologist even "blew out" his sinuses! All reports were negative.

Since no one could detect a disease process or any pathology, Mr. F.F. was advised his problems were psychosomatic; he was probably suffering from "insecurity in the high executive position he held at such an early age." He entered psychiatric therapy but soon stopped, realizing this too was futile.

One day, almost by accident, Mr. F.F. found that a cocktail seemed to relieve his headaches. A few drinks helped him to complete his work and to get through the day. He started drinking more and more, and by the time he first visited an optometrist, he felt he was becoming, in his own words, "an involuntary alcoholic."

Dr. William Ludlam's initial testing revealed a possible latent two-eyed problem; further intensive examination, including patching one eye, confirmed this. A special prismatic prescription was dispensed for him, along with some simple home vision training instructions. A few weeks later, Mr. F.F.'s headaches had completely disappeared. He was overjoyed at having found "a non-alcoholic solution."

THE HYPOCHONDRIACAL CHIROPRACTOR

Whenever Dr. R.B.W., a 52-year-old chiropractor, started to read or do close work, he felt the strangest sensations in his eyes; itching, burning, tearing, discomfort, and occasional pain would set in within thirty minutes. Over a number of years, these symptoms increased in severity to the point where he had to almost stop all near work.

He consulted several eye doctors. Each one gave him at least two pairs of glasses, but none of them helped. As time went by, Dr. R.B.W. began to think his problems were due to "nervousness." He wondered if the dizziness, the gastrointestinal disturbances, the abdominal cramping, and the all-over feelings of tightness and tension were imaginary. In desperation, he consulted numerous physicians, and even fellow chiropractors. Finally, he came to Dr. J. D. Bartlett, an optometrist, who made a positive diagnosis of aniseikonia. The appropriate prescription took care of this two-eyed problem, and he has felt well ever since.

The following is a letter of appreciation, written by Dr. R.B.W. to Dr. Bartlett:

> "I am extremely proud and happy to say that most of all the symptoms have disappeared in these sixty or so days I have been wearing this appliance. I don't believe ever in my life having sighted down a board, fence, or line or whatever you may care to use as an example, and found it to be true. It is amazing to me the new world that I have found of balance and truisms in lines and parallels.
>
> I am truly living in a new experience and I am thankful for it. Thankful for what I can see and what it has done for me in a physiological way, ridding me of many of the things which had begun to cause mental problems in my wondering what was wrong and why someone couldn't do something about it."

In trying to identify visual problems, or any health disorders and their systemic symptoms, it is important to keep in mind that they don't just happen. Symptoms do not exist in isolation but are *meaningful expressions* of some underlying disorder—warning signals for our conscious mind.

The mysteries of the neural and endocrine networks of the human body and their interconnections are only beginning to be revealed. Scientists are only starting to realize the true complexity of human functioning in general, and visual functioning in particular, and how the two are really one and the same thing.

The sufferings of our three friends brought about by their weak two-eyed visual systems can be likened to being in a constant state of conflict—a visual tug-of-war—for most of one's waking hours.

One way to decide if a particular symptom is two-eyed in nature is to remove one of the contestants from this tug-of-war, i.e., to patch one eye. Numerous case studies have demonstrated that the exclusion of one eye has often been the key in eliminating other chronic symptoms—symptoms that may have been previously thought of as psychological or non-visual in origin.

Symptoms of two-eyed struggling and the various forms of neurosis, depression, general nervous tension, anxiety, etc., overlap in many areas, so much so that true neurotic symptoms might actually take someone to the optometrist, while symptoms of binocular stress might take another person to the psychiatrist. For this reason, we believe that both specialties should understand each other better and cooperate more closely in investigating a possible link between mental and binocular instability.

The case studies we have presented, do not in any way represent the complete spectrum of visual complaints. The reader must bear in mind that a variety of different disorders may produce the same symptoms, just as any given visual problem can elicit different symptoms. It is the analysis of the constellation of signs, medically termed syndromes, and not the isolated complaint or test result that forms the basis of visual diagnosis.

Efficient two-eyed vision is not only a luxury but a great responsibility. The onus in seeking the best care available for its preservation, is upon you; the responsibility for the diagnosis of your particular visual problem should be the optometrist's.

SYMPTOMATOLOGY OF BINOCULAR STRESS

(An adaptation of Optometrist Dr. Raymond R. Roy's findings)

Many of the symptoms of two-eyed stress may parallel those arising from different bodily conditions.

- headache
- post cervical tension
- trapezius tension
- thoracic area backache
- hypersensitivity to light
- general nervous tension
- appetite loss
- nausea
- vomiting
- nervous stomach
- sleepy feeling

- insomnia
- motion sickness
- vertigo
- slow reading
- skipping lines
- one-eyed reading
- pulling on eyes
- conversational difficulty
- disturbed feeling in crowds
- hypersensitivity of skin (generally scalp – usually associated with severe headache)
- inability to remember previous conversations
- periodic blurred vision (often present in the early morning, shortly after awakening)
- frowning
- double vision
- depression
- sudden upward rolling of eyes with excessive blinking
- obscure abdominal pain

CHAPTER NINE

THE POWER OF LIGHT

MAN is a heliotropic organism, naturally attracted to light. We bend to light just like plants. Our eyes are light detectors. Light through its various focal positions triggers physical mechanisms in the eye and helps to create the psychological effects of different colors.

Imagine a see-saw with Blue and Red at opposite ends. Blue is known to be calm and content, and would be satisfied to sit and meditate all day. Psychologically and physiologically, Blue is at rest, counter-balancing the more energetic and nervous Red. If we relied on Blue's initiative, the see-saw would never get off the ground.

Red stimulates action; it is a physical color as opposed to Blue's spiritual qualities. Situated at the heat end of the spectrum, it is warming, sensual, and emotional, symbolizing the deepest of human passions—love, hatred, and courage. Red is energy-expending and just thinking of it will increase your blood pressure, heart rate, and respiration.

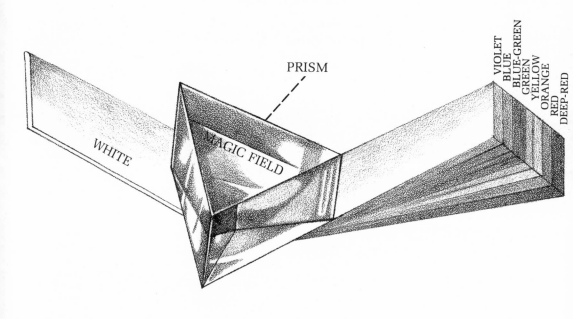

I'm colorless, drab and plain dull, complained White.
I need a new friend to make me feel bright.
And so White asked Prism to make him glow,
Together they found, White had color to show.
As White passed through the Magic Field
The rainbow colors he did yield:
Deep-Red, Red, Orange, Yellow, Green,
Blue-Green, Blue, and Violet were seen.

Let us move on, to gain further insight into the physiological secrets of light. Due to lack of color correction in the human eye, white light entering your lens will be broken up (refracted) into the same spectral positions, just as it was after passing through the prism.

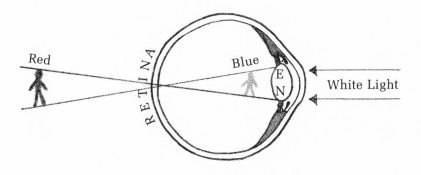

This is a cross-section of the human eye.

This is another see-saw with Red and Blue on opposite sides, but this time the fulcrum or pivot is your retina, the photo-sensitive element at the back of your eye. Any light precisely focused here would give you 20/20 eyesight. This is quite a static state.

Can part of this evolution of color-associated, social phenomena be related not only to the inherent nature of the color but also to its interaction with the human eye's focusing system?

Red, which focuses behind the retina, will appear blurred to the eye, and must signal the brain to focus it in. Now Red becomes clear, although it had to work hard to do so; by its very focal position, it is a stimulus to that all-important focusing mechanism of the human eye.

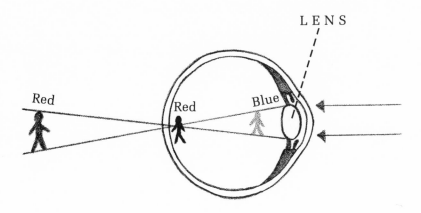

Positive focusing or accommodation is allowed.

Red is analogous to the far-sighted individual whose eye lens also focuses light behind the retina. In order to see clearly, the far-sighted person must be constantly active to keep the focusing mechanism at work. Hyperactivity, general restlessness, and short attention span can aptly be associated with Red and the far-sighted individual.

Light, such as Blue, which focuses in front of the retina, will also be blurred. But Blue has no recourse; under normal conditions, the human eye lens cannot focus negatively.

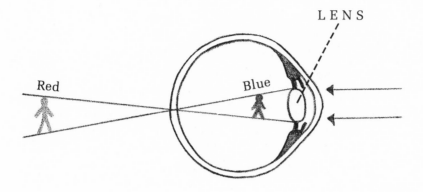

Negative focusing or accommodation is not allowed.

Under blue light, the focusing system is, in a sense, deactivated. Since things are blurred, many near-sighted people, are more prone to sit and think. Let us look at the development of the near-sighted personality from another perspective. Could its more introverted nature have developed out of a need to put the focusing mechanism to rest? Or can its near-centered nature be related to the physiological factor, that the near-sighted individual has reached a state where he or she need not focus as much as those with "normal vision?"

Kirlian photography, or field radiation photography, gives a visual representation of the internal energy state of the human being—the human aura. Russian studies show that different sections of the skin, under normal conditions, characteristically emit different colors; under different physiological and emotional states, the colors seem to change. It is interesting that a characteristic state for good health and relaxation is a blue-white corona. This normal, blue-white corona changes to a red blotch when the person is in a state of tension or anxiety.

Alpha waves, electrical rhythms from the visual area of the brain, induce a state of psychological and physiological calm. Thousands of people have sought to reach a higher level of awareness through control of these waves. In humans, these waves are best produced when the eyes are closed. When the eyes are open and focusing normally, alpha waves are suppressed. Experiments have shown that the blue region of the spectrum is considerably more effective than the red region in activating or photically driving the alpha waves.

What practical application does our knowledge of light have for us? We should be able to coordinate the lighting and color schemes of our near working environment for the benefit of our color-oriented focusing systems. Special hygienic lighting rules will allow children to develop their as yet fragile, accommodative systems.

Any source of light not properly coordinated, received either directly from a lamp or reflected indirectly from walls or a desk, will draw us away from a visually near-centered task. Dr. D. B. Harmon has shown that we tend to reflexively center our bodies in the brightest spot in our surroundings. A poorly contrasted light environment will provoke a tug-of-war between undivided attention to a task and our naturally phototropic tendencies. The traditionally brown school desk therefore sets up a high contrast between the task and the working area, causing a visual fixation conflict between the edge of the task (book) and its details (words).

A difference in illumination of as little as 12 per cent between the two eyes will result in a disturbance of two-eyed vision. Have you ever noticed someone shut one eye in bright sunlight? This could be an indication of a breakdown in two-eyed vision due to different light distribution; it emphasizes the significance of the directional position of task-incident light.

There is much controversy concerning the exact intensity of illumination necessary for optimal learning efficiency. Dr. D. B. Harmon maintained that there is no such thing as an exact amount of light suitable for each task, that "illumination levels needed for resolution of all aspects of a task are variable functions of the details of the task, of patterns of brightness in the visual field, and of achievement demanded in performing the task. Studies have shown that the finer the details in a task, the more light is needed, and the higher the level of achievement demanded, the more light the individual tends to require." In general, if the lighting is too strong, the visual ability to function will decrease due to glare of various kinds; if the lighting is too weak, resolution of detail becomes difficult, setting up undue stresses in the visual system. To determine the general illumination required for a particular task, let *comfort* be your chief guide.

The following are recommendations for a visually conducive, luminous working environment. We have adapted most of the rules from Dr. Harmon's book, *The Coordinated Classroom.*

- The most visually efficient working surface should be of clear finish, light, natural wood with a light asymmetric woodgrain pattern.
- Background colors in ceiling, walls, and floor should be desaturated, grayed or warm white, but not drab, to prevent the influence of unwanted color on the focusing system of your eye. The wall you are facing while you work is especially important in this regard.
- The contrast relationship between the task (book, paper, etc.) and the immediate surrounding surface should not exceed 1 to 1/3; i.e., if the brightness of the target is 1, the brightness of the surroundings should not be less than 1/3, nor more than 1.
- The ceiling should form the primary source of diffuse illumination. Spot illumination, such as a lamp on the desk or any other light at eye level, sets up unwanted contrasts and creates discomfort glare.
- Sometimes, a standing lamp can complement the diffuse room illumination. A helpful rule of thumb is to use a 200 watt lamp, 15 inches (38.1 cm) away from the center of your reading or working area. To prevent disturbing shadows, the lamp should be over your *left* shoulder if you are *right-handed* and over your *right* shoulder, if you are *left-handed.*
- Never work directly *in front* of or *parallel* to a window or with the window directly *behind* you.
- To overcome the adverse stresses produced by daylight in your near-working environment, rotate the

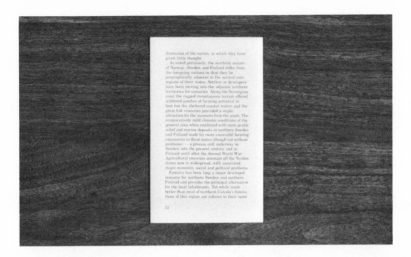

A high contrast is produced between the "school-brown" desk top (reflectance 13 per cent) and the visually-centered task (reflectance 70 per cent). There is a conflict in fixation between the edge of the task and its details.

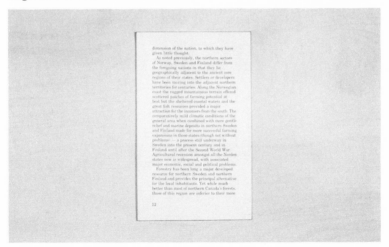

The same visually-centered task placed on a desk top of natural wood finish eliminates conflict. Task reflectance is now 70 per cent while desk top reflectance is 45 per cent. Note ease of fixation at any point.

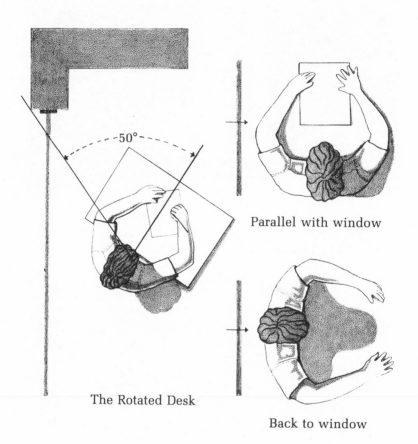

50°

The Rotated Desk

Parallel with window

Back to window

seats and working surfaces so that the farthest limit of the window which could fall within your visual field is 50° from the line of sight.

- Even though the sun is the best source of light for visually near-centered activities, it may create discomforting glare under the above conditions. If you feel bothered by sunlight, we suggest you draw the blinds and use the recommended artificial light.

THE SUNGLASS REVOLUTION

The Sunglass Revolution began during World War II when the United States Air Force needed a device to effectively protect the eyes of high-altitude pilots against glare. A green-yellow "anti-glare" glass was developed. Why green-yellow? Because it provided the nearest to normal light, resulting in minimal disturbance of color perception. Subsequent research into the benefits of outdoor filters revealed that to be most effective in bright sunlight, a sunglass "should exclude not less than 80 per cent of the whole light."

Like many new trends, the sunglass trend brought with it new problems. There are tints in exotic colors which are fine for fashion occasions but do not qualify for sunglasses. Misleading, glamor-ridden advertising brainwashes people into choosing fashion first, while optical considerations take second place. Unfortunately, most of these tints do not meet the 80 per cent absorption requirements of true sunglasses. It is the chemical ingredient in the lens and not the color that is responsible for absorption of harmful rays. This has several serious consequences, the most dangerous of which is inadequate protection

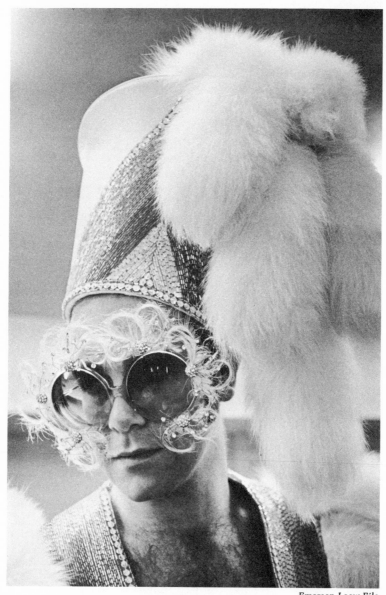

Emerson-Loew File

The Fantastic Elton John

against the rays of the sun. Prolonged exposure may result in possible tissue damage due to the harmful effects of invisible ultra-violet and infra-red rays which lie outside the visible spectrum of white. Over-exposure to sunlight through light fashion tints adversely affects night vision, making it hazardous to drive in the dark.

The goal of the original sunglass was to reduce glare while maintaining the constancy of color perception. Any degree of inherent color-blindness in the wearer compounds the adverse effects fashion tints have on color perception. Misinterpreting colors can be potentially dangerous when driving, operating machinery, etc., To check for color distortion, look through the lens at a white surface; it should be darkened but not appreciably colored.

The sunglass fashion trend also brought with it the hazards of poor quality and imprecisely-ground lenses. Irregularities found in these lenses can interfere with normal vision, causing distorted images, eye strain, fatigue, headaches, and nausea. The easiest way to check for irregularities in a non-prescription sunglass is to hold it at a little less than arm's length and look through one lens at a surface, such as a window, which has both horizontal and vertical lines. Move the lens from right to left and up and down. Any motion or wavering of the horizontal or vertical lines of the windowpane indicates a warp in the lens.

Everyone is buying plastic lenses nowadays since they are so much lighter than glass. Unfortunately, most plastic lenses, regardless of color, do not filter out the infra-red part of the spectrum. Thus, under conditions of prolonged exposure to bright sunlight, wearing plastic lenses may do you more harm than good.

Here are a few hints for sunglass wearers:

- Wear them only under conditions of prolonged exposure to glare.
- Never wear sunglasses indoors except under professional advice. Continued indoor wear will make you even more sensitive to light (photophobic).
- Don't wear sunglasses at night. They substantially reduce the already dim illumination and can be outright dangerous.

The organic point of view maintains that the ultra-violet rays should *not* be totally excluded from entering your eyes, as a full spectrum composition will have a positive effect on your health and disposition.

Colored lenses, windowpanes, fluorescent, and other artificial lights, all distort the natural spectrum. However, there is a full spectrum, plastic (organic) lens, termed neutral gray, on the market. Unlike ordinary sunglasses, it effectively reduces *all* wavelengths of light over the visible and invisible spectrum but cuts out none, thus keeping the balance of natural sunlight. Color perception also remains unaltered. These full spectrum, plastic, neutral gray sunlenses are manufactured by Armorlite Inc., 130 North Bingham Drive, San Marcos, California, 92069. They are available throughout the world. (In Canada, the distributors are Imperial Optical Company of Toronto, Ontario). Ask your eye doctor about them.

Our entire nervous and endocrine systems are influenced by full spectrum, natural light. While the skin is generally thought of as the intermediary organ in terms of health, research has revealed that light entering the eye can also contribute to normal body functioning. We mentioned earlier that about 20 per cent of the visual fibers are posturally linked and do not go directly to the visual cortex. There is another group of visual fibers that through the neuroendocrine system influences the powerful pituitary gland—the master gland—which in turn controls the adrenal, sex, and thyroid glands. Natural light can thus profoundly influence hormone production throughout the body.

Our luminous, artificial lighting environment distorts the spectrum of natural sunlight. It has been found that people who work constantly under artificial light suffer from a number of physical and mental disorders. John Ott, a noted light researcher, discovered that dental caries and hyperactivity in children are triggered by radiation given off by fluorescent light. His experiments point to the possibility that certain types of cardiovascular diseases and cancer may actually be promoted by artificial, polluted lighting. In contrast, Dr. Ott maintains that, in some instances, human cancer and various other ailments could be beneficially influenced by full spectrum light, and that the time may not be far off when light will be prescribed as a form of medical and psychological therapy. A full spectrum, fluorescent bulb is already being used in hospitals in the United States and in Canada. This bulb can provide the benefits of natural light indoors. In the United States and in Canada, Vita-Lite is obtainable under the Duro-Lite label in the indoor plant section of department, hardware or lighting specialty stores. Commercial installations are handled by Duro-Test Inc., North Bergen, N.J. in the United States, and in Canada by Duro-Test Electric Ltd., Rexdale, Ontario. The manufacturer reports that children working under this purer type of artificial light demonstrated increased alertness, did more and better work, and developed greater resistance to fatigue. According to the Industrial Electrification Council, " ... efficiency, welfare, behavior, and happiness are dependent upon light and vision; ... good lighting helps keep down absenteeism, encourages promptness, and steadier employment ... "

Until the Industrial Revolution, people spent a lot of time in natural light. Since then, most of us have been forced to pass much of our days behind walls and windows of office buildings, schools, homes, etc. Walls exclude natural daylight altogether, while windows distort it in different ways. One of the negative effects of window glass and conventional, artificial light, is the almost total filtering out of ultra-violet rays, so important for the manufacture of Vitamin D. We recommend the installation of full spectrum, plastic windows in homes and offices. Rohm & Haas Co. in Bristol, Pennsylvania and its Canadian subsidiary in West Hill, Ontario manufacture this type of plastic window which is available through their distributors. (For other manufacturers and distributors of plastic sheets, check your local directory.)

Ordinary prescription glasses also exclude ultra-violet light. With this in mind, we recommend Armorlite's special, full spectrum, plastic lens. Again, ask your eye doctor about it.

Car windows, like any other window glass, absorb the ultra-violet rays which are necessary to activate the new photochromic lenses. As these lenses automatically darken outdoors in sunlight, they will be relatively ineffective inside a car and therefore for driving.

Light is our behavioral director, emotional determinant, metabolic stabilizer, and life supporter. There is no doubt that the nature of the luminous environment we have created for ourselves has profound physiological, psychological, and social effects upon us. The future promises enormous possibilities for our well-being if we effectively learn to control this environment.

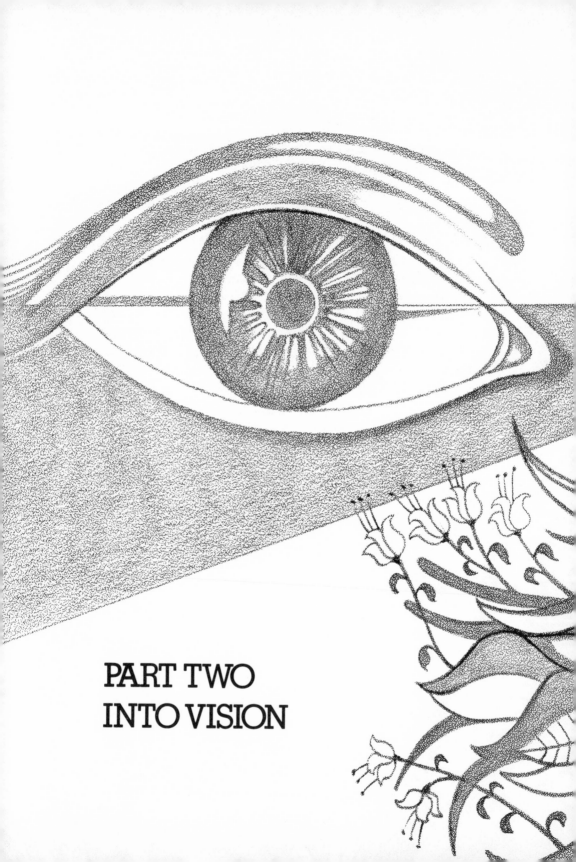

PART TWO
INTO VISION

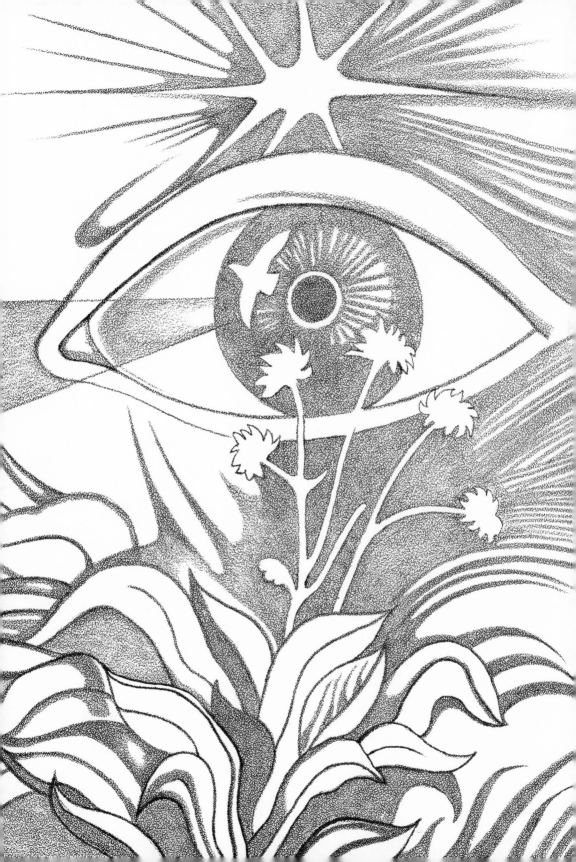

CHAPTER TEN

MOVEMENT, SPACE, AND VISION

YOU are surrounded by space from the moment you are born. Every movement you make is a movement through space. You are having a spatial experience every second of your waking life. However, you had to learn how to organize these movements and how to deal effectively with the space that surrounds you.

Imagine yourself submerged in a world made of honey. Your movements would become slow; you would have to learn to operate and visually guide yourself through a new medium, as all around you strange forces would exert pressure on your body. Your movements would meet with resistance; you would encounter restraint and try to fight against it.

Movement through space is the key to visual growth and development. At birth, you only have sight, not vision. You see but you do not understand. In order for vision to emerge, you need all the sensory movement experiences you can get. A consistent relationship between body movement skills and vision movement skills has to be firmly established. Only when seeing begins to coincide with doing, can vision adequately substitute for and become independent of movement.

This process of learning to see starts within arm's reach. At this distance you first learned to *see* and *feel* your hands at one and the same time. It was here, in near space, where the seeds of your vision were planted, where visual understanding began with, "where is it? – what is it?" and was then extended one step further into distance space. Movement, therefore, appears to be the first stage in understanding space. Seeing and doing must be slowly translated out of near into far space, as distance vision becomes an extension of near vision.

The organization of self, the inner space, must precede the organization of outer space. How can you be expected to successfully interact with the outside world and its demands if you have not yet mastered your own world of feelings? You must first become aware of the parts of your body, of your relationships, your schemata and how to control them in order to reach an equilibrium with your own environment.

A significant portion of the nerve fibers from the eye do *not* go to the seeing areas of the brain but are involved with the balance and postural mechanism of the body. Vision is therefore a total process which utilizes the head, the neck, and the trunk for orientation in space.

Stand up in a relaxed position with your head erect and arms thrust forward, parallel to the ground. Balance on your toes while looking at some distant point for a few seconds. Now shut your eyes and you will experience the effect vision has on maintaining balance. Vision is balance!

As the relationship between vision and movement matures, we should rely less and less on our motor skills and more and more on our vision skills, until vision ultimately dominates and movement becomes subservient. We now have the privilege of becoming observers without first becoming participants.

Vision, as it substitutes for movement, helps to steer, guide, and refine movement, to predict and appraise its results, and to record its consequences. This process sets the stage for the development of communication patterns (speech, language) to replace action.

Vision helps us understand the things we cannot touch, taste, smell, or hear in near or far space. We can even transcend physical barriers of time and space and be thrust into the fourth dimension of abstract thought.

You can fly,
High as a kite if you want to,
Faster than light, if you want to,
Speeding through the universe.
Thinking is the best way to travel.

This space odyssey points out the most basic aspect of the vision developmental schema: how you have built your "space world." You first had to learn to understand yourself in order to establish a successful rapport with your environment. Insight into yourself and your movements leads to visual thinking, visual judgment, foresight, communication, and ultimately visualization, the symbolic translation and reconstruction of reality—to "see in the mind's eye." At this ultimate stage of visual development, you have truly emerged OUT OF SIGHT INTO VISION.

CHAPTER ELEVEN

A CHILD'S
CONQUEST
OF SPACE

AT a very young age, children have no real conception of space. Their visual judgments are poor guesses in their, as yet, unformed world. Unsophisticated, clumsy, and awkward, they grope and drag themselves hesitatingly through the space that surrounds them. It is as if they were submerged in the honey we spoke of earlier, with forces crowding in from all directions. Their visual fixation pattern is still under-developed.

The next time you see an infant in a crib, try this: pick up a small, shiny object such as a bell and slowly move it across the baby's field of vision, from side to side, and up and down. Notice how the infant picks up visual fixation for a moment, only to quickly lose it again. The baby may actually try to reach for the bell; it is as if the hand were the extension of the eye, vainly struggling to reach and grasp the object.

If you see one eye turn in or out momentarily— don't be alarmed! At this young age, from birth to eighteen months, the visual sense is still crude and operating on a primitive level. Babies are prone to eye

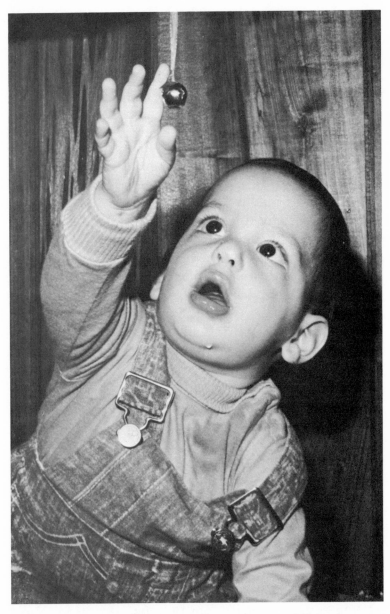

It is as if the hand were the extension of the eye.

turns as they lack complete organization of either side of their bodies and it is, therefore, not surprising that they have poor two-eyed vision. Their lack of internal organization is further reflected in a randomly generated body pattern and a non-purposeful behavior that is almost exclusively motor.

Compared to the infant, the child between the ages of two and three-and-a-half will have a better concept of space. Behavior remains unorganized but in this age group a child can put a puzzle together although he may take a long time to complete it. Notice the use of the same hand to hold and manipulate the pieces while the other hand hangs limply. Behavior is purposeful for only one side of the body. Movement and touch play the primary roles in exploring space. Vision is secondary, as small children appear to be using their hands to see.

At this age, young children are frequently distracted by peripheral signals in their environment; the noise of a car speeding by the window, a glimpse of mother or father out of the corner of the eye will attract their attention and pull them away from whatever they are doing.

They are also head turners, as if they could not move their eyes without moving their heads. In whatever they do, they invariably tilt the head a little, tap one foot, or open and close the mouth. These unproductive movements are essential for their performance; we call them "motor-overflow."

Two-eyed vision is only partially functioning. With regard to spatial judgment, there is a significant difference between the two eyes, as the child still struggles to see. With limited spatial outlook, how can he be expected to turn right or left when there is no body concept of right or left? How can he be expected to follow directions? At this stage, all performance relies heavily on movement with vision in support. Behavior may be aptly described as "motor-visual."

Once a child reaches an age of between four and six, he has built a fairly efficient spatial world for himself and is better organized and a lot more competent than the previous age group. If you get a chance to observe a five-year-old playing with a puzzle, you might see that both his hands are involved in the task. Although both sides of the body are now operating, movements are not yet fully integrated. Vision has become the primary sense in the perception of space; movement and touch provide reinforcement to visual judgment and have become secondary. These children are using their eyes to see, their hands to refine seeing. They will alternate the right hand with the left as they have not yet built up one side that dominates. They will also alternate central with peripheral regard; one moment they are seemingly intent on the puzzle, the next they are looking out of the window, yet are able to return quickly to their tasks.

Two-eyed vision operates well with some inefficiencies; concerning spatial judgment, there is a mild difference between the two eyes. Try the bell experiment with a child in this age group and notice how the eyes pick up fixation easily, the head moving as if in support. Although each eye sustains fair control and attention, seeing still requires some effort.

This child can follow directions as she has developed a better concept of her own right and left

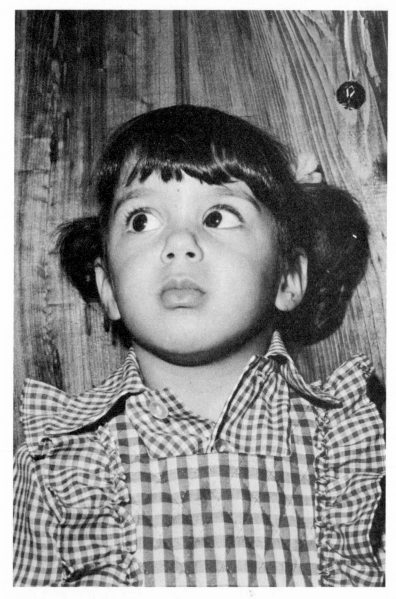

Children in this age group are frequently distracted by peripheral signals.

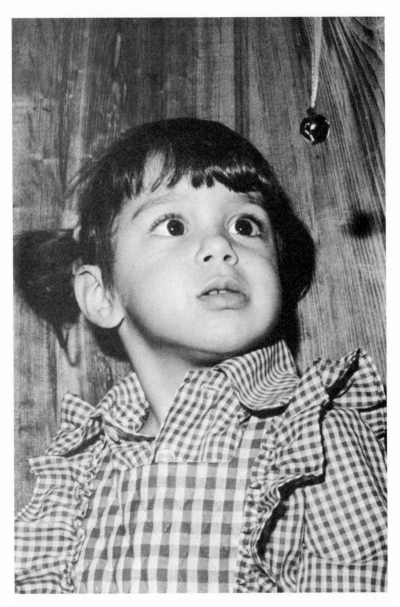

It is as if they could not move the eyes without moving the head.

side. Her self-image enables her to project internal awareness of both sides of her body into three-dimensional space. This type of behavior, where visual sense leads and directs and movement supports, is termed "visual-motor".

When a child reaches the seventh or eighth birthday, we can expect the space concept to be well developed. Behavior is purposeful and goal-seeking, and tasks are executed with complete integration of both sides of the body. Vision has replaced movement in space to become the primary sense through which space is evaluated. In piecing together a puzzle, both hands operate and act competently in a lead-support fashion; based on visual judgment, the pieces are the right way up before they are placed in the puzzle. One

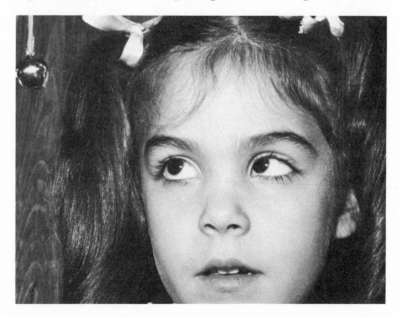

Her eyes pick up fixation easily while her head moves as if in support.

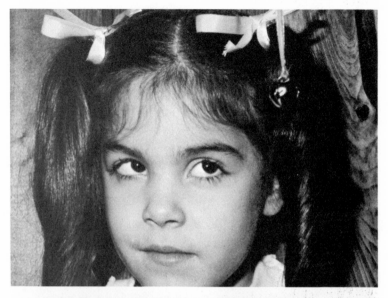

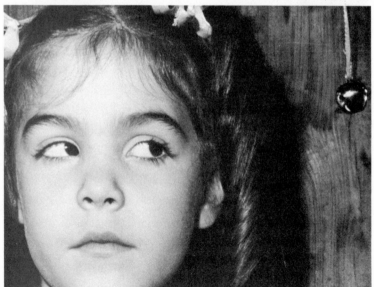

Although each eye sustains good control and attention, seeing still involves some effort.

hand fits the pieces in place while the other confidently feeds them to the hand that fits the pieces. This child has effectively bridged the gap between the right and the left side of his body, and is no longer in a trial-and-error situation. Unproductive motor-overflow has been eliminated and the central-peripheral relationship is entirely balanced and fully consistent. The child can function well in his own space world, free from all but the most disturbing stimuli, and is able to focus attention for long periods of time on a puzzle or on any other near task, while maintaining peripheral awareness.

This is the coordinated child who makes the right turns at the right times. He has developed a good sense of directional awareness, knows where to go and, more importantly, when to go. He has no problem to reach, to grasp, and to release visually. To follow the bell, no excessive head movements or supportive head turns are required. This child will move his eyes without having to move his head while he reads, as each eye sustains complete control and attention. He can handle all visual tasks with rhythmic coordination and accuracy. There is no difference between the two eyes with regard to spatial outlook, as seeing has become an effortless joy! At this stage, your eye doctor will likely tell you that your child has good two-eyed vision—full binocular function. Thus, visually satisfied, your child has become a truly visual human being!

The visual-motor hierarchy we have described follows a normal developmental sequence:

Motor—Birth to 1$^1/_2$ years

Motor-Visual—2 to 3$^1/_2$ years

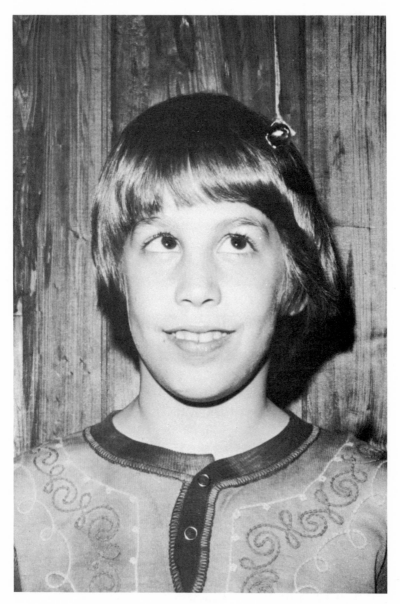

A truly visual human being! Seeing is an effortless joy.

Visual-Motor—4 to 6 years

Visual—6 to 8 years

Just as you had to learn to use one hand at a time, you also had to learn to use one eye at a time. Only when you were able to use both hands and both sides of your body in a truly integrated and purposeful manner, could two-eyed vision be expected to operate effectively. "During early life, while developing the ability to control parts of self first, then of self and the world, it should not be surprising that, in some cases, the part begins to operate *as if* it were the unitary whole! When this happens, a developmental deviation results." (Dr. John Streff, Optometrist). The eye turn is one of the most prevalent, developmental deviations. As much as 90 per cent of crossed eyes set in before the age of five. In these cases, the one eye often tends to dominate and operate singly as if it were the *whole* instead of just *one half* when making visual judgments. This is part of the development of the "lazy eye syndrome."

A child who experiences difficulty putting body and eyes together will have difficulty matching seeing with doing. If one eye turns, the information received will conflict with the information gained, not only from the other eye but also from the other senses. Confused and in a turmoil, the child is forced to seek a way out: he gives up the use of one eye. In a sense, by doing so, he has adapted well to the situation compared to the individual who still operates with an inefficient and weak two-eyed system. The "one-eyed" person's problem is less obvious and will become apparent to all but the one who has fragile, weak, two-eyed vision.

Our eyes are structured to provide two types of vision–central and peripheral. By focusing in, our central vision acts as an "attention-holder," a lock. Our peripheral vision is more sensitive to movement and shapes *around* the object of attention, and keeps us aware of happenings around us; it is important for our survival. In a manner of speaking, our peripheral vision is the *vigilante* of our central vision. Only in the last stage of the visual-motor hierarchy, can these two systems operate in a truly balanced fashion. A consistent central-peripheral relationship, is the epitomy of stress-free, efficient seeing.

Many problems arise if two-eyed vision operates on either the central or the peripheral wavelength. Directives are available to help remediate these problems early in life, and may be carried out at home, if supervised by a vision specialist. The following is an adaptation of ten directives taken from the Infants' Vision Clinic of the University Optometric Center:

SPECIFIC HOME GUIDANCE FOR BINOCULAR PROBLEMS

1. Between the ages of three months and one year, patch the eye for 2 to 3 months as directed:
   a. First day: right eye completely covered
   Second day: both eyes open
   Third day: left eye completely covered
   Fourth day: both eyes open
   b. Other, if indicated.
2. Place the child's crib in such a way that the window or greatest light source is on the same side as the deviating eye.

3. Whenever the parent feeds, plays with, or hands things to the child, it should be done from the same side as the deviating eye. As much activity as possible should take place on that side.
   a. *If the eye turns in* – a central type of seeing pattern – more efforts should be made to approach the child with toys and other stimulation from the back as well as from the periphery (far side) of the turned eye.
   b. *If the eye turns out* – a peripheral type of seeing pattern – more efforts should be made to approach the child with toys and other stimulation towards the center of the body, so that the child can grasp the toy or react to stimuli with both hands.
4. The child should be encouraged to creep. Avoid the use of a playpen as it tends to restrict creeping. To discourage walking, place the child on an inclined mattress or board.
5. Lift the child by both hands or lift him as he clings with both hands to a bar or a broomstick handle.
6. Have the child roll or toss a lightweight, oversized ball to make him use both hands at the same time.
7. Toys should include large building blocks, nesting toys, color cones, etc.
   a. Have the child stack them.
   b. Encourage him to pick up a block and bring it to you.
8. Encourage the child to play with large push toys, such as a wheelbarrow, that can be moved with both hands.

9. Play peek-a-boo, covering the good eye for brief moments.
10. The older child should be encouraged to jump onto and off a one inch (2¹/₂ cm) thick board, raised approximately two inches (5 cm) from the floor.

Passing through the various visual-motor stages is not an automatic process; if its normal sequence is disrupted, developmental vision problems may occur. These do not only affect children; you yourself may, at this very moment, demonstrate some signs of passing through an immature stage in your own visual-motor hierarchy.

CHAPTER TWELVE

THE DEVELOPMENTAL VISION PROBLEM

GROSS-MOVEMENT in space is a prerequisite for perceptual development; eye movement is necessary for visual perception. The image of a stimulus presented to a stationary eye would fade. To insure this perception, an invisible, physiological tremor of the eye is required to slightly alter the instantaneous presentation of the stimulus. We are able to piece together a meaningful picture of our spatial environment through fixation movement. Light stimulates the retina, the photo-sensitive element at the back of the eye, and causes a movement response. Visual movement triggers body movement. These motor responses are monitored through vision, which can guide, record, and ultimately predict them.

If we reflect on the interdependence of vision and movement, we realize how visual skills are but motor expressions of human performance. This theory is a far cry from the primitive concept that sight is sensory or that sight may be sensory, but vision is motor!

Of all our senses, vision is by far the most efficient critic of space. A child, retarded in visual-motor development, would have difficulties understanding space. If that child is not able to correctly project directional concepts into space, he may have difficulty perceiving the difference between the letters "b" and "d", and may not be able to comprehend words which denote spatial positions, such as *up, down, in, out,* etc. A visual problem will result from interference with the orderly developmental processes of vision, usually triggered by deprivation and/or restriction of movement in space during early childhood.

The two main interacting factors, space and movement, combine to produce the following equation:

Restrained Movement

+

Restricted Space

=

Developmental Vision Problem (D.V.P.)

generalized:

Lack of Sensory-Movement Experiences

+

Interference with Development of the Space World

=

Not visually ready to be taught (D.V.P.).

R.C. Orem, in his book *Learning to See, Seeing to Learn*, cites common, everyday examples of environmentally restrained movements in space, based on parents' comments concerning their infants' behavior:

"He was such a good baby, never gave me any trouble; all I had to do was set him on the floor and give him a few toys, only a few, and he never moved away from that same spot until I picked him up; he never cried and was very satisfied to stay put."

This child never learned to use both eyes simultaneously. He alternately used his right eye or his left eye, when doing a near-visual task. When he looked far away he used only his left eye, and ignored his right eye.

"We know what you are looking for, we have studied the pictures in the baby book; they show that we have always held him the same way, in the left arm with the right side of his face against our bodies, so that he was always looking up with his eyes turned to the right when he looked at us; we never held him any other way."

The child lacked visual experience in looking to the left and ultimately developed a crossed left eye.

"The floor was too cold, so we always kept him in the playpen; at least he was not underfoot when I was trying to do my housework, and I knew where he was if I wanted to read a book or watch television."

Not given the opportunity to learn how to use both sides of his body, this child's eyes did not work well as a team. Body and eye movements were erratic and inaccurate.

"I did not put him in the high chair except at meal-time; he started throwing things when he sat there and wore me out picking them up. I then just stopped giving him toys when he was in his high chair. If he started throwing his food, I took it away until I had enough time to feed him."

The child was deprived of necessary muscular and visual experiences to adequately judge distances in space.

"Our bedroom was so small that the crib was always in the same place, over by the wall." (When Optometrist, Dr. D. McCoy inquired whether the baby was ever shifted in the crib, the mother asked, "Why? should he have been?")

This child did not receive equal and balanced visual stimulation of both eyes since one eye was always "locked" into the wall. He was found to be using one eye only for distance and near, and never developed the use of both his eyes.

None of the children in the above examples developed adequate visual abilities.

Sensory-movement activities that should help your child "learn to see" include experiences in handling a variety of textured and/or differently shaped, objects and puzzles, doing finger and brush painting, building with blocks, or stringing beads. Hopping, skipping, jumping, climbing up and down steps, target throwing, and rope jumping, are equally valuable exercises. A more comprehensive list of activities is provided at the end of this chapter.

It has been shown that rearing a very young child in a drab, uniformly colored, and restricted environment will adversely affect not only his visual, but also his general perceptual development. To help your child get a good start in life, we put forth the following suggestions:

- Keep a small, dim light in your baby's room at night. This will not only help placate him but will give him visual stimulation, so necessary to learn the most basic skill of fixation.
- Change your baby's position and that of his crib at various intervals to allow the stimulation of light, e.g. from a window, to come from different directions.
- Do not use crib liners as they will block your baby's view and can "lock him in" visually.
- Use colored, printed crib sheets to provide patterned light stimulation; colored pictures and designs hung on the wall or from the ceiling of your baby's room are additional sources of visual stimulation. A homogenously colored visual field, such as a blank white wall, stimulates the retina but carries no other information. Hang balloons, brightly colored pieces of paper, and mobiles well above your baby's crib to hold his visual interest.

Tragically, many young children are entering school not visually mature. The problem is compounded by educational authorities who often lack awareness of this fact. Every child should be examined for visual readiness before entering kindergarten. Proper grade placement might eliminate as much as 50 per cent of the difficulties children experience in school, according to Frances Ilg, M.D., former director of the Gesell Institute of Child Development and Louise B. Ames, Ph.D., Director of Research at the same institute. This is important because the child's problem may be a simple lack of maturity versus actual retardation in development. Frequent progress checks are essential to insure adequate learning. Visual awareness is enhanced by play programs which incorporate activities such as those mentioned in this book. If further activities are indicated for your child they should be prescribed by a vision specialist.

Better testing programs are urgently needed. The antiquated 20/20 concept of vision falls short in detecting readiness problems and lags in visuo-motor development. A developmental vision problem is usually noticeably present by age 5, and the stress of first grade serves to compound it. The aware teacher and/or parent can readily pick up signs of these problems. Here are some of them which point to possible visuo-motor lags or visual immaturity:

- Child's head turns as he reads across the page;
- vocalizes when reading silently;
- needs a finger or marker to keep his place on the page;
- writes crookedly and/or spaces poorly and cannot stay on ruled lines;

- has poor general body coordination;
- rejects hand-eye activities;
- must feel things to assist him in any required interpretation;
- repeatedly confuses left-right directions;
- confuses likenesses and does not notice minor differences;
- fails to visualize what he has read, silently or aloud;
- confuses letters or words;
- reverses letters or words;
- squirms, fidgets, and is hyperactive.

An "Educator's Checklist of Observable Clues to Classroom Vision Problems," prepared by the Section on Children's Vision Care and Guidance, Optometric Extension Program Foundation, Inc., is reproduced at the back of this book. Copies of the "Educator's Guide to Classroom Vision Problems" may be obtained from any Clinical Associate of the Optometric Extension Program Foundation. Copies of the Checklist *only* are also available.

Visuo-motor training is not simple. For this reason, we shall not attempt to lay out an actual developmental program. Also, a child who has difficulties at school may have a host of other problems which might require a multi-disciplinary approach.

As a concerned parent or teacher, understand vision, space, and movement; know what to look for! You will be better equipped to take the appropriate steps to seek out remedial care for a child with a developmental vision problem.

BASIC SENSORY-MOVEMENT ACTIVITIES FOR CHILDREN

At an early age, your child's visual process must be integrated with all his other sensory and motor systems. To assure proper visual development, Dr. E. Forrest and Dr. D. Fitzgerald, of the Infants' Vision Clinic at the University Optometric Center in New York, have worked out the following basic sensory-movement activities:

General
- Whenever possible, talk, sing and play with the child.
- Allow the child time for play and exploration by himself.
- Avoid the restraints of a playpen, crib, and high chair during those periods of the day when they are not required. Let the child move around as much as possible.
- Show affection to the child.
- Try to approach the child from different sides, at different times. This goes for feeding or playing. It is also recommended that the crib be moved to different positions of the room on different days, if possible, so the child will not always face the light from the same side.

Eye Movement Abilities
- Hold a flashlight or penlight before the child and move it from right to left, left to right, up and down, diagonally, and in circles while talking to the child as he tries to follow the light.

- Shine a flashlight at a wall and move it slowly while the child tries to follow the beam visually.
- Play flashlight tag with the older child by having him hold his own flashlight, while trying to follow the beam of yours with his.
- Play "airplane" while feeding the child, by circling the spoon in the air, and making a buzzing sound as the spoon approaches his mouth.

Hand-Eye Coordination
- Stacking blocks.
- Nesting blocks.
- Block building.
- Stringing beads.
- Tossing and catching balloons.
- Closing the fist and opening it one finger at a time.
- Ring toss.
- Push toys.
- Pull toys.
- Take-apart toys, as well as percolators and kitchen utensils.
- Peg or nail pounding.
- Follow-the-dot games.
- Folding and unfolding napkins.
- Modelling clay or play dough.
- Tossing bean bags at someone or into a basket.
- Simple puzzles.
- Tracing and coloring.
- Free painting or finger painting.
- Tracing around wooden, plastic, or cardboard forms. Using large crayons or coloring chalk on a chalkboard placed on the floor, and later against a wall.

- Spreading food in front and to both sides of the child as he eats.
- Having the child switch a small object from hand to hand, while he puts on a shirt or sweater.
- Placing pegs in a pegboard.
- Dotting O's in a newspaper or telephone directory.
- Coloring and filling in drawings.

General Movement and Balance Skills
- Setting up an obstacle course composed of chairs, tables, hassocks, and boxes in such a way that the child has to crawl under, over, and squeeze between narrow obstacles.
- Playing "take 1, 2, or 3 giant steps; take 1, 2 or 3 baby steps."
- Pushing a wheelbarrow.
- Holding the child's ankles as he becomes a wheelbarrow.
- Walking backwards.
- Toe touching.
- Running games.
- Peeking through legs.
- Jumping from steps or blocks.
- Balancing on one foot.
- Hopping on both legs.
- Hopping on each leg.
- Stepping on cracks.
- Laying a rope on the floor and letting the child jump over it.
- Rolling, throwing, bouncing balls.
- Sit-ups, push-ups, etc.
- Walking on a "walking rail", 8 foot, 2″ × 4″ (2½ m, 5 × 10 cm)

- Balancing on a balance-board.
- Tapping hands and feet, 1. RH, RF, LH, LF. 2. RH, LF, LH, RF.
- Crawling and creeping.
- Ball bouncing.
- Playing hopscotch.
- Tossing and catching balloons.
- Rolling a ball.

Body Concepts and Self-Imagery

- Exposing the child to the concepts of front-back, up-down, big-small, side-side, and one-two, in terms of body parts.
- Using a floor-length mirror and having the child watch himself as he moves different body parts on command.
- Drawing around the child's hand or foot, making an outline. Having the child match the drawing with his own body parts by pointing to the big toe, the little toe, the thumb, etc.
- Teaching the child to touch on command your head, hair, shoulders, stomach, hand, foot, leg, arm, neck, mouth, ears, eyes, chest, back, fingers, etc.
- Teaching the child to touch his own body parts on command.
- Playing in a sandbox, making imprints of body parts (feet, toes, knees, hands).
- Playing poem games, such as:
  "Hold both hands up;
  open them, shut them,
  open them, shut them,
  give a little clap;
  open them, shut them,

open them, shut them,
put them in your lap."
- Playing "Hokey-Pokey":
"Put your little arm in . . .
put your whole self in . . .
put your *right* hand in . . .
put your *left* foot in . . ."
- Playing "What" games.
What sees? (eyes)
What hears? (ears)
What smells? (nose), etc.

Communicative Ability

- Tracing designs in the air while the child tries to guess what they are. Having him do the same for you.
- Following simple directions: stand up, sit up, close the door, open the door, come here, etc.
- Imitating sounds: How do we laugh? (Ha, Ha, Ha). How do we sneeze? (A-choo). How do we whistle? How do we cough? etc.
- Pantomine: Pretending you are a soldier, a police officer, a cat stretching, a circus acrobat, a baseball player, an elephant swinging his trunk, a dog begging, a baby crying, a horse galloping, a flower growing up, up, up, then down, down, down; pretending you are bouncing a ball, sweeping, mopping, peeling potatoes, driving a car, etc.
- Singing while the child acts out the song:
"This is the way we wash our clothes, wash our clothes, wash our clothes. This is the way we wash our clothes, early Monday morning."
Then, "this is the way we iron our clothes; mend our clothes; stir a cake," etc.

Auditory Awareness

- Blindfolding the child, or having him turn away from you. Making the following noises and having the child identify them. Crushing paper, whistling, knocking at a door, tapping on glass, writing on a chalkboard, blowing on a harmonica, clapping hands, drumming, playing piano; imitating noise-makers, pounding, coughing, running, jumping, snoring, crying, walking, etc.
- As the child progresses, have him try to identify: money jingling, blowing into a bottle, scratching, rain falling, leaves rustling, paper tearing, paper-bag popping, etc.
- Having him identify whether the sounds he has heard are high or low, near or far, loud or soft.
- Imitating animal sounds, and having him identify a bee, a dog, a cat, a bird, a horse, a pig, a duck, etc. Having him imitate these sounds for you.
- Having the child imitate sounds heard on phonograph records.
- Singing rhythmical songs such as "London Bridge," "Mulberry Bush," "Ten Little Indians," etc.
- Having him clap hands to a beat.
- Tapping to a certain number of beats, and having the child repeat them back to you.
- Telling stories to the child.

Intersensory-Motor Discrimination

- Sorting and counting objects.
- Identifying coins.
- Blowing different-size soap bubbles.
- Taking a quick look at an object and identifying it.
- Learning colors, using colored balls or blocks. In

stories emphasizing the colors of objects (red wheels, blue dress), while pointing to something that has that color. Having the child find the red block, the yellow crayon, the brown belt, the green lollipop, etc.

- Hiding a button in one hand. While both hands are closed, asking the child to guess which hand holds the button.
- Playing with shadows on a wall.
- Making felt puppets for hands and fingers.
- With the child's eyes closed, placing some food or drink in his mouth while he tries to guess what it is.
- Repeating this exercise using various odors.
- Introducing the child to different objects by having him close his eyes and try to distinguish the objects by touch. Examples: cotton, sandpaper, felt, paste, smooth stone, rough rock, shiny paper, sand, pencil, doll, toothbrush, key, leaf, wood, etc.
- Teaching directions and space relations, by having the child move his arms in and out, up and down; by walking towards and away from something, by climbing under and over something, by turning left to the window and right to the door, by planting seeds and watching them grow.
- Encouraging the child to discriminate between objects which are *heavier*, *lighter*, or those which make more or less *noise* when dropped, by using a paperweight, a rock, a brick, cotton, paper, a block, a feather, a book, a tin can with and without sand, a balloon, a stone, etc.
- Encouraging the child to discrimate between small objects and large ones (ball, box, etc.), as well as between tall and short objects (doll, bottle, etc.)

- Having the child learn the *names* of objects, by asking: "Show me the _____! Where is the _____? Give me the _____! Put the _____ into the box!" (ball, airplane, wagon, chair, table, bed, door, window, coat, scissors, apple, etc.)

Distance-Oriented Games

- Throwing a ball into a basket or a large box, moving the receptacle farther away as the child achieves success.
- Throwing a ball at specific targets across the room.
- Throwing a bean bag at a drawing of an animal with its mouth open.
- Playing "Hit the Penny" with a large ball.
- Throwing a ball into a hula hoop, first held in the air and then left resting on the ground.
- Calling the child's attention to and discussing objects that are at a distance.
- Playing "Catch," moving further away as the child improves.
- Pasting different pictures on a beach ball, having the child roll the ball across the room, telling you what picture is facing him when it stops.

CHAPTER THIRTEEN

SENSIBLE
SEEING

A **MAJOR** theme of this
book is based on our contention that in today's society
social and environmental demands force us into virtually unacceptable situations biologically. The restrictive learning, working, and leisure environment
into which we are thrust daily, frequently prevents or
tends to break down the development of our natural
seeing patterns.

These acquired, and often faulty patterns may
lead to physical and mental warps, i.e., actual structural changes in the body with resulting perceptual
skews. You bend to adjust to the environment
whereas the environment should bend to adjust to
you. To enable you to tune into the correct visual
wavelength, and gain maximum benefits from the
light energy that surrounds you, you must develop a
proper outlook, a new level of awareness, and acquire
a seeing pattern that is free and easy.

Your working environment can be physically
constructed with hammer and nails in your own

home, where you study or play, or whenever you or your child engage in near, visually-centered activities. The study area, especially, must have its own sense of understanding and built-in appreciation of your visual systems—an area that will work *with* and not *against* you.

Your own particular perceptual mode can be mentally constructed. Since vision is a learned, developed function, it is trainable. It would be nice to be able to build a little awareness circuit into your own system, one which would effectively process visual information.

The significance of a physically conducive learning environment has been amply demonstrated by Dr. D. B. Harmon's classic study at the Becker School in Austin, Texas. In the fall of 1942, the school was rearranged and coordinated to conform with certain criteria to allow maximum freedom of performance at minimum physiological expense to schoolchildren. Six months after the classrooms were reorganized, it was found that visual problems had been reduced by 65 per cent, nutrition problems had dropped by 47.8 per cent, and signs of chronic infection had been reduced by 43.3 per cent. In addition to the improved health of the children, some comparable results in educational achievement were also obtained.

Using the following examples, we shall try to help *you* arrange some of the conditions, originally conceived by Dr. D. B. Harmon.

EXAMPLE 1:

Pick up this book; you are undoubtedly holding it at an angle, when you begin to read.

For physical hygienic reorganization of your near working environment:

Rule: Use a tilt top desk.

Purpose: To create a balanced posture for near-centered tasks.

Theory: Reading material, correctly angled, to complement a normal reflexive position, will reduce energy expenditure in the entire body.

The traditional use of flat top desks in schools and homes creates visual image distortions, sets up adverse stresses in the system, and decreases efficiency when processing information. By jutting the desk top into space we are, in a sense, giving a 3-D quality to a 2-D task. We strive for dimension in our visual world; we shun flatness. Stereopsis, or 3-D vision, is the epitomy of two-eyed vision. If however, the near-centered task involves a 3-D activity to begin with, i.e. modelling or block building, a flat top desk is needed.

Apparatus: A 20-degree tilt top desk can be easily made by screwing two door stops to the back of a piece of plywood and two rubber knobs to the desk to prevent the plywood from slipping.

EXAMPLE 2:

While reading, how far from your eyes are you holding this book?

Rule: For near-centered tasks use the *Harmon Distance*, the distance from the middle knuckle of your fingers to the center of the elbow, measured along the outside of the arm. It is the minimum distance at which close work should be done.

Purpose: The second step in creating a balanced posture is to set up a distance at which the two hands can interact efficiently with the eyes.

Theory: This distance is an important prerequisite for effective physiological functioning at near-centered tasks. It is anatomically unique for each individual and is based upon the measurement of working distances used by over 40,000 people with "normal vision." People under visual stress unconsciously tend to reduce their working distances.

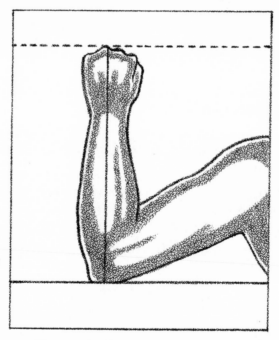

The "Harmon Distance" is the minimum distance at which close work should be done. It is measured from the middle knuckle of your fingers to the center of your elbow, along the outside of the arm.

Anyone intently bent over a near task, gives credence to the old saying, "to keep one's nose to the grindstone." We want to break this pattern and prevent your world from closing in. Many parents falsely attribute a child's contorted writing posture to bad habit instead of to faulty seeing. Have your child momentarily close both eyes while he writes. You may observe that he suddenly sits up. Vision and posture are closely connected.

EXAMPLE 3:

Where are you sitting now? Can you adjust your chair or desk? Are you reading in bed?

Rule: Desk and chair should be adjusted for correct height; chairs must be able to rotate freely, with back-and-forth play.

Purpose: This example creates a balanced posture for near-centered activities, and will allow a child freedom for growth.

Theory: Properly designed furniture that considers the reflexively assumed body position for near work will reduce energy expenditure in the entire body. You must be free to perform, free to maintain optical and motor relationships, while your pelvis is in a balanced position with minimum compression and restriction of soft tissues. A bucket-seat type of chair, with movement built into it, will accomplish this.

It is a fallacy that it is good to sit up straight in a chair, as to do so creates tension in the back muscles. Bend your back slightly. Reading and studying is a mental activity and fatigue is not only caused by eyestrain but also by the muscular effort required to keep the body in a prolonged sitting position.

Apparatus: The chair should be adjustable to the height of the desk so that with the upper arms hanging free, you should be able to slide your elbows on top of the desk. Chair contours should be those of a bucket-seat. The chair should be free to move forward, backward, and in rotation.

EXAMPLE 4:

Have you ever noticed your child having difficulty using a pencil? What about you?

Rule: Use a proper pencil grip.

Purpose: The final step in creating a balanced posture for near-centered activities is to improve penmanship.

Theory: Faulty seeing is not the only cause for contorted posture during near-centered activity. It can also be induced by an improper pencil grip. Gripping a pencil is a learned skill and a difficult developmental task to master. Far too many students grip pencils so low and so awkwardly that they block one eye's line of sight and are forced to lower and tilt their heads to see what they are writing. Writing becomes labored as the writer moves his whole hand, fingers firmly clenching the pencil. Poor penmanship, stressful eye focus, poor eye alignment, and bad body posture, can result in slower learning and a shortened attention span. When thumb, index finger, and middle finger gently grip the pencil about 1-1¹⁄₂ inches (2.5-3 cm) above the tip (a little higher for "lefties"), correct posture becomes possible. The eyes can function more naturally with less strain, and free and easy finger movements are allowed to develop in the writing hand. The forearm of the hand that writes should be parallel to the edge of the paper while the non-writing hand should act as support, holding the paper in place to prevent it from slipping.

Apparatus: A Posture Pencil Grip (GRIP-E-Z Gripper) developed by Hoyle Engineering Company, 302 Orange Grove, Fillmore, California 93015, is a vinyl, triangular grip that slips over the end of a regular pencil or pen. It is mounted one inch (2.5 cm) above the tip and cushions the writing fingers. These grippers are available from MacMillan School Supplies stores in the United States, and in Canada from the Association for Children with Learning Disabilities, 4820 Van Horne Avenue, Montreal, Quebec. Posture Pencil Grips will benefit everyone, but are especially useful for schoolchildren in elementary grades and those with learning difficulties.

THE FREE-HAND SQUARE TEST

The following test, devised by Dr. D. B. Harmon, demonstrates the possible relationship between the body balancing mechanism and visual performance, in near-oriented tasks such as reading, writing, and drawing. Initially devised for elementary schoolchildren, it can be used by people of any age, and is valid for anyone capable of drawing free-hand squares.

Write your name. Make three rows of squares as rapidly as you can, approximately the same size as your handwriting. Children should print their names in capital letters.

Evaluation of results:
- Rectangular squares will indicate that the individual is working *off* or to the side of his midline.

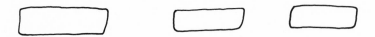

- Squares to the right indicate a head tilt and reflect an inability to align.

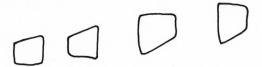

- If the product is readjusted along the line, or if there is a space break along the line, perhaps two to the line, the individual is a slow reader.

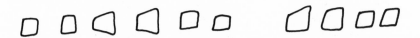

- Horizontal curves will indicate a head tilt, with the eyes not equi-distant from the task. If one vertical line is longer than another, this means an effort is being made to fuse two differently sized squares. This performance is related to unequal visual patterns in the two eyes, e.g., one eye is more near-sighted than the other, or one eye is near-sighted and the other is far-sighted.

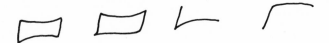

- The products below indicate a tendency (latency) for one eye to be higher than the other, combined with unequal visual patterns in the two eyes. This latent hyper-deviation generally induces visual differences between the two eyes.

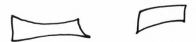

- The following product is indicative of suspensions (turning off the vision in one eye).

- Looking across the paper, with the head down and too close to the task will produce the following product:

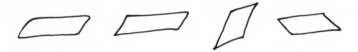

- A trapezoid (2: 1 width to height) is an astigmatic product. Astigmatism is a condition where light enters the eye forming line images instead of a point focus.

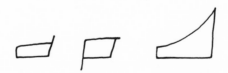

- Vertical tails closely correlate with a tendency for one eye to be higher than the other—low tails for high side and high tails for low side. In time, this individual will develop more and more atypical visual signs, not measurable by optical devices. Symptoms will appear in different regions of the body, e.g. as neck pains and occipital headaches, low back pains, and by the need to shift the weight to one foot while standing.

- Horizontal tails seem to be related to a two-eyed coordination problem, a tendency for the eyes to deviate either inwards or outwards.

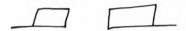

- Smaller than average squares indicate a myopic tendency; larger than average squares indicate a tendency towards far-sightedness. There is an 80 per cent chance of a myopic or far-sighted tendency when the product is either smaller or larger than the average size of the small round letters in your handwriting (2 to 3 mm).
- Wide spacing between squares indicates a tendency for the eyes to posture outwards, narrow spacing between squares indicates a tendency for the eyes to posture inwards.

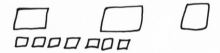

The above test will provide insight into your own unique visual pattern, without necessarily disclosing a visual problem. The results become clinically significant only in combination with a complete vision analysis.

CHAPTER FOURTEEN

SEEING
WITH
AWARENESS

BY breaking adverse seeing patterns you will also break adverse working patterns. If you do not focus or channel your visual energy effectively, center or converge your eyes properly, of if your *outlook* is segmented and inconsistent, your thought process will likely be inconsistent and frequently irrelevant to your situation. The result will be a state of visual vacancy: "Being without seeing; thereness without awareness."

Persons searching for a name in a building directory, selecting a song in a juke box chart, or reading items on a menu, are performing tasks which disseminate a lot of visual information. Someone who lacks the flexibility to align the eyes and think at the same time might find himself staring blankly at the building directory, standing in front of the juke box while others restlessly wait in line or, having looked at the menu in a restaurant for about ten minutes, that person might be "awakened" by the waitress, and say: "Oh, I haven't decided yet."

We would like to help you cultivate a sense of

awareness. People seek many ways to attune their bodies to the world around them. They do it through yoga, meditation, the martial arts, or through exercise. We shall try to give you the means to do it through vision. It might sound mystical but there is really nothing mystical about getting in tune with your own feelings, or in touch with your own body through vision. Vision is the major link between outer and inner space. Three million impulses enter the brain every millisecond, two million of them go into the visual area!

We believe increased awareness is the culmination of vision training. The techniques we suggest should be part of a daily routine and are not meant to replace professional training for the remediation of visual problems. Some of these techniques were designed by the University Optometric Center and have been adapted by us. These simple, visual hygiene exercises and rules, apart from leading towards intuitive awareness, may:

- prevent a breakdown in your visual pattern;
- halt deterioration in your visual skills;
- improve the functions of an already intact visual system.

We have included body calisthenics to be used in conjunction with visual calisthenics. By mastering both, a truly positive mind-body relationship should result.

VISION TRAINING EXERCISES

Before attempting prolonged near work, such as reading, typing, needlepoint, or painting, we recommend you try this visual warm-up, as an integral part of your daily exercises.

Exercise 1   Stand six or seven feet (1.75 to 2 m) away from a wall, without your glasses on. Keep your head absolutely still. Look at the upper left corner of the wall for about three seconds; then shift your gaze to the upper right corner for another three seconds. Repeat, looking at the lower right corner; then the lower left corner of the wall, to complete the cycle. Do ten cycles clockwise and ten, counter-clockwise. If you experience stress in any position of gaze, don't force yourself to continue, work slowly.

This procedure is the first step towards breaking out of an undesirable, overly central, seeing pattern. It helps loosen the eye muscles, especially those that move the eyes into different positions of gaze. It directs your vision into those areas of space where you might have difficulty looking and propels more oxygen into your visual system.

We have mentioned *looking out*. This referred mainly to looking out in one direction – straight ahead, looking beyond – to relax focusing and to prevent the world from closing in. But we can look out in more than one direction – out of the corners of our eyes, to the left of us, to the right of us, above and below our normal line of sight – while looking straight ahead.

This is *peripheral* vision. The amount or field of peripheral vision can be clinically determined. How *much* peripheral vision you have is one thing, how *well* you use it is something else. We call this the quality of peripheral vision, peripheral and environmental awareness or, simply, the "awareness factor." Individuals may possess clinically intact peripheral vision, yet, at the same time, bump into objects constantly, in a typically clumsy fashion. These individuals have a poor visual grasp of the spatial layout necessary for their efficient locomotion.

Because we use our peripheral visual system for the detection of movement, it plays a major role in our survival. When you see a car speeding down at you, you see it first out of the corner of your eye (peripheral system). Assuming you are not looking directly at it, an eye movement is reflexively triggered to alert your central vision. Only a lightning reaction will save you from an accident.

The ability to utilize peripheral vision selectively for processing information is the zenith of peripheral awareness. To achieve the ideal of sustained central attention, while maintaining peripheral awareness, necessitates a balanced relationship between the peripheral and the central visual systems. Some near-sighted people, by warping their visual patterns, develop a preoccupation with central detail; they are "locked in." Physically, they tend to operate in restricted space, with inhibited body and eye movements. Visually, they "focus in" on detail but suppress and become less aware of surrounding details. Psychologically, they become introverted with a limited "outlook."

The following exercise is designed to help increase your awareness and create a better balance between your central and your peripheral seeing.

Exercise 2   Sit on a couch in your living room or in

any other place where objects are all around you. Fix your eyes on a point in the room. Think of nothing else but that point; maintain your awareness. If it happens to be the knob on your stereo set, you are probably aware of the stereo set and one or two objects around it. Now, look out farther and farther, always keeping your eyes on the knob. Increase your awareness of the objects immediately adjacent to the set. Continue to look in an arc-like fashion, imagining yourself in the center of the arc. Become aware of the objects to your right and to your left in an ever-increasing arc, as if they were in orbit around you. Slowly, add one detail at a time, first one on the left, then one on the right. Although you do not have eyes in the back of your head, try to visually *feel* the space behind you, while you remain aware of the objects within your field of vision. This will help increase your perceptual field.

Hold that image and begin to increase your awareness of the rest of the room. Start in a vertical direction, keeping your eyes on the knob. What is above it? Be aware of it. What is below it? Be aware of it. Look diagonally. Fill in the entire space of the room. Be as "far-sighted" as possible. Repeat this exercise in different situations in another room, outdoors, etc.

To develop peripheral awareness in near space, use the following clinical optometric technique devised by Dr. Lawrence Macdonald. The goal is to expand the amount of visual information that may be comprehended, per given unit of time.

Exercise 3 Occlude one eye with an eyepatch. Hold the Form Recognition Field, 13 inches (33 cm) away

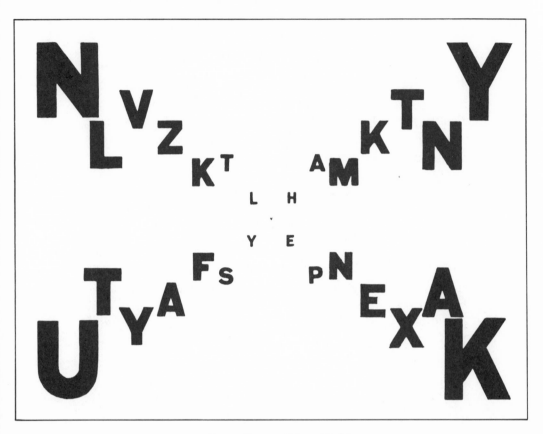

Form Recognition Field

from the other eye. Your posture should be relaxed and easy; keep your body as still as possible. Fixate the center "v" at all times. Try to recognize the four letters immediately surrounding it. If you cannot recognize these four letters, shift your gaze to one of them, possibly the H, and gradually move back to the central "v" maintaining recognition of the H. Continue in the same manner with the next block (T A P S) of four letters and then the next, until you have achieved peripheral perception of the last block (N K Y U). Now try to visually grasp the first block of four letters all at once, then eight letters all at once, and so on. The ultimate goal is to be aware of all the letters at the same time. Try and see these letters as clearly as possible, while keeping the center "v" clear. Vary the technique by varying the distance between you and the Form Recognition Field from between 9 and 20 inches (23 cm and 51 cm). Repeat the exercise with the other eye, then with both eyes without the eyepatch.

To assist in transferring this activity to space and general living, continue to look at the "v" in the center. Observe the other letters out of the corners of your eyes using your peripheral visual function. Do the letters appear to remain still? Does the apparent blackness of the letters seem relatively constant? Try to see all letters simultaneously. To help relax your body, try and make the field appear homogeneous and steady, and try to see the total field at once.

When you can see most of the letters simultaneously and homogeneously, look to the space in front and around you. Try to maintain the same feeling of homogeneity and simultaneity. Observe any area in relation to the total space; that is probably the way space exists out there. Each area is as important as every other, occupying its own space in relation to all other space. Try to see it that way.

Exercise 4   The following exercise is to build peripheral awareness, one eye at a time. Obtain six 3 × 5 inch (7 × 12 cm) white index cards. Draw 2 inch (5 cm) high numerals, 1 through 6, in the center of each card. Fasten the six cards to a wall in the following manner: cards 1 and 2, 12 inches (30 cm) below the ceiling, separated laterally by about 72 inches (1.75 m); cards 3 and 4, 12 inches (30 cm) above the floor and separated laterally by about 72 inches (1.75 m); cards 5 and 6 are centered between the two sets. The diagram illustrates the positioning of the cards:

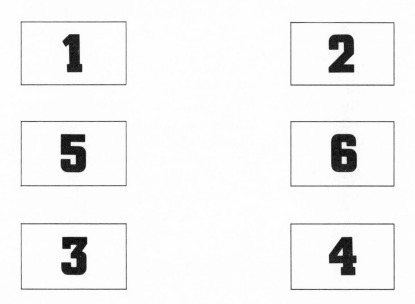

Stand 72 inches (1.75 m) away from the wall, centered between the cards. Without exerting pressure, cover one eye. Keep your head as still as possible. Look at card 1 at the same time as you try to become aware of as many of the other numbers as possible. While looking at card 1, you are using your central visual system; your peripheral vision should perceive the other cards. Without losing awareness of the number on the original card, switch your gaze to one of the other numbered cards. Remain aware of as many numbers as possible. Repeat the procedure with the other cards, then start all over again, using the other eye. Peripheral *awareness* of the numbers on the cards means awareness only; it does not mean 20/20 discrimination.

Remove all but one card from the wall and keep it at eye level. Move to within three feet (1 m) of the wall. Cover one eye. Attach a small coin to a pencil tip and have someone bring it slowly into your peripheral field of vision. The pencil should be held vertically at the opposite end, flat against the wall. Keep your gaze centrally fixed on the number on the card. Your head must stay absolutely still all the time. Your eyes will tend to wander away from the center towards the periphery. Your friend must not let you do this. Signal when the coin first comes into your peripheral field of view and mark the spot on the wall with a piece of tape to gauge your progress. Repeat this for the whole circular field of view, converging from eight directions—two horizontal, two vertical, and four diagonal. Repeat this test for the other eye. The aim is to increase your field of peripheral perception. To further enlarge the field, imagine seeing the coin before it actually comes into view.

General calisthenics, especially those involving the neck region, will ultimately prove beneficial to the visual system. Movements of the body relieve stress and strain and induce a relaxed state of mind which, in turn, encourages the visual system to relax.

The following two exercises are stress-reducing techniques. The feedback between the skeletal system and the external eye muscles will also help offset postural warp tendencies. Both exercises are best done for about five minutes at a time, *after* prolonged near-centered activity.

Exercise 5   Take off your glasses. With your eyes open, slowly rotate your head in a rhythmical, circular motion, making sure your eyes follow the direction and the full extent of the rotation. Your eyes should follow your head; feel your eyes and neck stretching. Do not strain; move your head slowly, first clockwise, then counter-clockwise, then vertically, horizontally, and diagonally.

Exercise 6   Stand upright in a relaxed posture and loosely swing both arms simultaneously forward, backward, and diagonally across the front of your body. Then, in a golf-swing manner, move both arms in a circular pattern before your body, first clockwise and then counter-clockwise.

The ability to change focus quickly and easily, looking from near to far, and from far to near, is one of our fundamental visual skills. It is necessary to build flexibility and to maintain a degree of freedom in our focusing system in order to better handle stressful visual demands. Inefficient focusing may cause vision discomfort and blurring at near or far.

Presbyopia, the reduction of focusing ability after forty, is a normal physiological phenomenon. The following procedure is valid for people under forty who still possess good accommodative focusing ability.

Exercise 7   Wear your glasses for this exercise. Construct an occluder mask out of cardboard (see diagram). At eye level, post a section of the day's newspaper showing the headline at a distance of approximately 20 feet (6 m). Hold the small print portion of the newspaper in one hand, approximately 16 inches (40 cm) away from you. In the other hand, hold the occluder mask in front of your face. When you look up, you will be able to see the large print with one eye, while the other eye will be blocked by the mask. When you look down, you should be able to see the small print with your other eye. Read the newspaper headline aloud for ten seconds, then look at the small

Occluder Mask

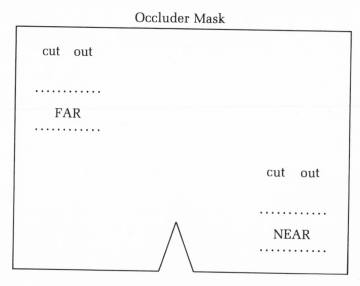

print for another ten seconds. Repeat this exercise for about one minute.

Now move the small print section of the newspaper closer, to about 8 inches (20 cm) from your face. Your goal should be to read the paper at this distance, without the print becoming blurred. If it does blur at any point, or if you feel yourself straining unduly, move the paper back to an area of clear vision and again begin to read. Reverse the mask and repeat. Exercise each eye no longer than five minutes.

To develop the ability to move your eyes smoothly and without effort, the following activity requires good coordination between the six *movement* muscles of each eye; you depend on this skill during all of your waking hours.

Exercise 8   Stand erect in a relaxed posture. Cover one eye with your hand on the same side. The other hand is thrust out—elbow straight, fingers gently clenched, thumb erect—to a point directly in front of your nose. Look at your thumbnail and move your arm in a circle, following your thumbnail with your eye while your arm rotates smoothly and easily. Do this three times clockwise and three times counter-clockwise. Repeat from side to side, up and down, and diagonally. Move only your arm and your eye, keeping your head still. Consciously release all tension. Work slowly. As you develop this skill, increase your awareness of other objects in the room. Repeat for the other eye.

Exercise 9   Another technique to develop flexibility in eye movements may be practiced with the use of a tennis ball hung from the ceiling on a string. Draw a number about 1 inch (2½ cm) high on the underside of the ball. Lie on your back with the ball suspended about 12 inches (1 m) above your chest. Look at the number on the ball while you keep your head absolutely still. Cover one eye and have someone set the ball in motion. Track the ball while it swings horizontally, vertically, diagonally, and in a circle. repeat this exercise with the other eye and then with both eyes.

If you experience unusual difficulties performing any of these exercises, you may have a visual problem and we recommend you seek professional advice.

VISUAL HYGIENE RULES

These rules have four basic functions:
1. to prevent your near working visual apparatus from going into a spasm;
2. to accentuate peripheral awareness;
3. to prevent eye and body fatigue;
4. to help maintain the delicate balance between central and peripheral vision.

Rule 1 Indoors or outdoors, with your eyes open wide look *towards* an object not *at* it. Become conscious of the background of the object. This will prevent you from directing all your visual energy to one specific spot in space. Masters in the martial arts (kung fu, karate) look *beyond*. By looking at an object in a defocused, non-central way, it seems to assume a more powerful and controlled image.

Rule 2 When you are outdoors, make it a habit, from time to time, to sight objects in the distance at about eye level, while becoming aware of the location of things in space all around you.

Rule 3   While you walk, especially in crowds, keep your eyes moving. This prevents your vision from becoming locked into your own body, as if your eyes had made a complete about-face in their sockets. Visual centering must be directed outward into space to keep your visual and thinking patterns alert and productive.

Rule 4   When watching television place the set at eye level, at a distance at least ten times the width of your screen. Anyone, who watches at excessively close range, may require professional visual analysis; near-sighted people have a tendency to develop this habit.

Do not watch in a dark room. To avoid glare and reflection from lamps, windows, or other light sources in or near the screen, the American Optometric Association recommends soft, overall illumination together with proper set placement. Brightness and contrast controls should be adjusted to individual taste *after* the proper room lights have been turned on. To eliminate visual distraction during television viewing, the area surrounding the set should be neutral in color.

Keep your eyes moving across the screen; do not let them remain stationary. Avoid looking up or down at the picture. Be conscious of the background of the set, and while you concentrate on a specific segment of the screen, be aware of surrounding space.

To relieve tension take a "visual recess" now and then, e.g., by looking out of a window, away from the set. Sustained viewing can lead to unnatural focusing and convergence fatigue.

Rule 5　Never read in bed, on your stomach, or in a moving vehicle, please! Be aware of space between yourself and the page, as well as of things around you, beyond the book. Occasionally, look out of a window at a specific object in the distance, possibly at a tree, until its details come into focus. Maintain awareness of other surrounding objects and details. This visual relaxation procedure should be done at least at the end of every two pages of reading. Also, place a bookmark every four or five pages ahead. Then get up and move around for at least one minute each time you reach the bookmark.

Never place your desk against the wall, as you will be visually "locked in" when you look up.

DISTANCE VISION TEST

On the inside jacket we have reproduced an eye chart which can be used to test distance vision for adults as well as for children.

Pin up the chart at a distance of 12 feet (3.6 m). Before testing your child's vision, teach him/her to point in the four directions without help. Use your three middle fingers to simulate the letter E, or reproduce the big letter E on a separate piece of paper for demonstration purposes.

By doing the exercises, activities, and tests we have suggested, and by following the rules we have outlined, you will be paying a small price in your attempt to achieve better and more efficient vision.

CHAPTER FIFTEEN

VISION
AND
YOUR BODY

THE existing relationship between vision and posture has been affirmed by many doctors for some time. Exhaustive studies by eminent men in pediatrics, physical medicine, ophthalmology, optometry, and education have expounded the concept that vision is a total bodily process, including its psycho-physiological and functional aspects. The concept is currently being utilized in the resolution of various vision problems.

THE TURNING EYE

Since vision is an integral part of human functioning and performance, we cannot think of visual distortions such as strabismus (eye turns) as divorced or separate from the total human being. Different doctors who treat strabismus are aware of and are taking advantage of the established relationships between vision, posture, and motor coordination. Chiropractors, for example, claim to have straightened turned eyes by postural adjustments to the back and neck. The team of Doman and Delacato, one specializing in physical medicine and rehabilitation, the other in education, have demonstrated that creeping and crawling activities at an early age are beneficial to strabismic children. Dr. A.M. Skeffington, an optometrist and former director of the Optometric Extension Program, told of children's crossed eyes straightening while they were creeping or climbing monkey bars. Other optometrists reported total elimination of strabismus in retarded children, following "neurological organization training" which included bilateral (two-sided) gross-motor activities. Dr. Bissaillon, another optometrist, after testing fifty strabismic patients, many of them infants, has described some of the bilateral activities he used in treating them. The infants, whose general physical coordination improved, usually became binocular while, with some exceptions, those whose general physical coordination did not improve, remained strabismic. According to a recent review of pertinent optometric literature by optometrist Dr. Martin H. Birnbaum, it was concluded that strabismus is frequently a local manifestation of a general lack of coordination.

In the same study conducted at the University Optometric Center, Dr. Birnbaum explored possible relationships between strabismus, gross-motor coordination, and postural deviations; he found that 50 per cent of strabismic patients tested showed foot posture deviations. About a quarter of these strabismics also demonstrated head tilts, shoulder tilts, and other bodily warps. Dr. Birnbaum concluded that "strabismus cannot simply be considered a turning of an eye with suppression and perhaps amblyopia (lazy eye). Results suggest that strabismus is an organismically pervasive condition and that we might speak of a *strabismic individual*, one of whose characteristics is an eye that deviates."

The University Optometric Center is a teaching clinic. It was founded in 1956 as an outgrowth of the optometry clinic of Columbia University. In 1971 it became the affiliated clinical institution of the College of Optometry of the State University of New York. While working at the Center, we observed how many strabismics functioned as if their particular problem also manifested itself in other areas of behavior: they were strabismics from the top of their heads to the bottom of their feet. For example, if their eyes tended to turn outwards (exotropia or walleyes), their feet would often display outward turns with a characteristic wearing down of the outer rim of their shoe heels. Conversely, if their eyes tended to turn inwards (esotropia or crossed eyes), they were often "knock-kneed," and their feet turned inwards (pigeon-toed).

As divergence excess strabismus is a common form of exotropia or walleyes, we noted how many of the children with this problem also exhibited other behavioral and visual traits. The most common, often first seen by parents, was the outward turning of one eye whenever the child was daydreaming, not paying attention to a particular task. When alert and concentrating, his eyes frequently appeared properly aligned. This condition was observed so often that the phrase "strabismus of inattention" was coined. Some of these children were academically hindered, depending to what extent their condition affected their

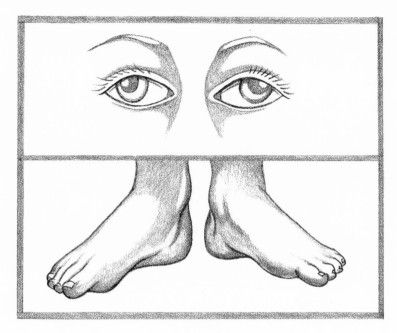

Exotropia

near space world. Interestingly enough, even though their eyes were turned out at distance, they often appeared straight or had a tendency to turn in, at near.

Children, whose performance was affected by divergence excess strabismus, could read well enough, as long as they read *slowly*. Attempts at speed reading seemed to adversely affect their visual patterns, with a corresponding drop in comprehension and frequent loss of place. They would complain of feeling tired and sleepy, and became careless and sloppy. According to optometrist Dr. Nathan Flax, these were the "streak hitters" of the elementary schools, the children who never found their middle

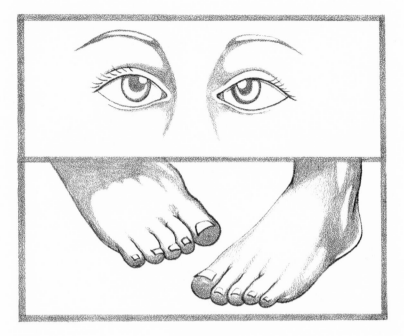

Esotropia

ground; they could either perform a task slowly and well, or quickly and sloppily. It seemed as if focusing, or the lack of it, was the core of their problem. When asked to *look in* and touch objects, a task which required fine and accurate focusing, their eyes would often *turn in*. It was amazing to see how strongly the tactual/kinesthetic sense was linked with and affected their visual performance.

Other tests confirmed that lack of focusing played a major role in the etiology of walleyes, a factor often tragically overlooked in the surgical treatment of this common visual problem.

Focusing, or too much of it, seemed to be at the

root of many of the crossed eyes we saw at our clinic. Focusing is linked with convergence. When this linkage is strong and inflexible, very often the result is too much focusing, accompanied by too much convergence. The eyes start to turn in and if this process is allowed to continue for a long time, the result can be an obvious crossed eye.

When we treat an individual for crossed eyes, we look for the underlying cause. If over-focusing is the only one, a simple *relaxing lens* will take care of the condition. Often this problem is compounded by anxieties, near-point stresses and emotional tensions. Linked with the autonomic nervous system, any increase in activity could well affect focusing. If an underlying emotional problem is present, we refer the patient to appropriate professionals.

Not every case of strabismus is due to focusing. There may be malfunction of the extra-ocular muscles, trauma, and congenital defects. It should, however, be stressed that congenital eye turns are quite rare.

Don't think a child will outgrow eye turns. Procrastination in seeking professional care allows complications to develop which will make it more difficult to treat the original problem. Keep in mind, there are rare instances when a crossed eye could be a blind eye due to a life-endangering tumor.

THE HAZARDS OF SURGERY

Early vision training attempted to make the two eyes work together and regain fusion; in strabismus, fusion is absent. It was often thought a weak muscle was causing one eye to turn in or out. Research has now shown that the extra-ocular muscles are over *one hundred times* as strong as they need be to perform their task. In fact, only about five per cent of eye turns are due solely to weak or faulty muscles.

It is the control of the muscle that is important. Unfortunately, in modern surgery muscles are often cut. Eye turns are regarded as anatomical phenomena. A traumatic approach to strabismus through surgery frequently causes multiple complications. According to the paper, "Mortality Related to Ophthalmological Surgery", statistics reveal that 0.7 per 10,000 American children still die from strabismus surgery today. Dr. I.M. Borish, the eminent optometrist and author of *Clinical Refraction*, comments that "a patient may have to forfeit life in undergoing optional strabismus surgery when other safe methods exist for strabismus remediation. This statement may seem shocking to some, but such occurrences have been regularly recorded for some time. The usual cause of death in strabismus surgery, as in other types of ocular surgery, is from cardiac arrest, caused by the so-called oculocardiac reflex."

Some authorities note that slowing of the heartbeat rhythm (bradycardia), which accompanies pressure on the eyeball, is inevitable in certain types of strabismus surgery; in some instances, it has been suggested to have been a cause of fatality in operations of this type.

In cases where visual training is not successful, we emphasize that surgery is only *one step* in treating *some* strabismic children. However, without further vision therapy, surgery alone is usually not successful as it only approximately straightens the eyes. Even if they seem to have responded well to the operation by appearing straight, focusing ability may yet be impaired, eye movement restricted, and sensory fusion may still be absent.

Although the initial operation is quite short, requiring only a few days' stay in hospital, frequently a second, and even a third operation may be necessary to achieve the desired cosmetic results. An extreme case in point is that of a girl who had strabismus surgery performed eleven times. The last operation left her with a marked eye deviation and constant double vision.

Complications arising from strabismus surgery include compensatory head tilts and body torques, post-operative pain, unsightly redness and the presence of scar tissue; occasionally, newly created ocular pathologies and infections may occur. In addition to these side effects, psychological and educational problems could surface. Dr. Reudemann, an ophthalmologist with many years of surgical experience, stated that unless appropriate vision therapy is administered after surgery, "we were developing our own group of neurotics, our own group of people who had nervous breakdowns, and people with inferior intellectual abilities."

SURGERY VERSUS VISION TRAINING

A glance at the success rate of surgery versus modern vision training shows that non-surgical methods not only have higher rates of initial cure but that success is much greater in the long run. In the article "Orthoptics and Visual Training" optometrists Dr. Martin H. Birnbaum and Dr. I. Greenwald state that "varying degrees of success in surgery for strabismus have been reported by ophthalmologists. Berke found that only 23 per cent of 256 patients with deviating eyes developed stereopsis (binocular depth perception) after surgery. Mulberger and McDonald report that surgery produced straight eyes and binocular vision in 11 per cent of 147 patients with eyes deviating outwards. Huggert studied a group of 105 patients with esotropia (crossed eyes), and found that 83 had no binocular vision after surgery. Kennedy and McCarthy in 1959 reviewed the results of surgery for esotropia in 315 patients. They found fusion (binocular vision) was produced in only 10 per cent of the patients.

"In contrast, Dr. William Ludlam, former researcher at the New York Optometric Center*, conducted a four-year study on the effects of orthoptic training upon 149 strabismics. He found a rate of cure of 77 per cent. This cure included individuals with functional and cosmetic binocularity. Furthermore, a follow-up study of these patients, three to seven years after completion of training, revealed that over 90 per cent had successfully maintained normal binocular vision." In a later study, reported in 1969 by optometrists Drs. Leon Hoffman, Allen H. Cohen, Gary Feuer, and Ivan Klayman, an overall success of 87.1 per cent of cure was achieved.

The following "before and after" photographs from the archives of Drs. Leon Hoffman and Allen H. Cohen who practice at Lake Ronkonkoma, New York, demonstrate the results obtained through applied vision training with strabismic children.

---

*Name officially changed in 1975 to University Optometric Center.

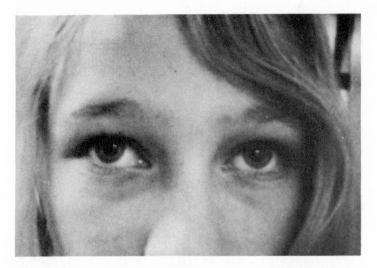

Before

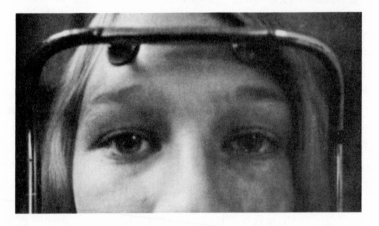

After

Patient 1 At age 13, Sandy showed moderate, intermittent exotropia with symptoms of occasional double vision, and constant closing of one eye. She also showed signs of eye strain when doing close work. Surgery was recommended for her condition. After six months of optometric visual training Sandy's eyes were straight and she was functionally cured.

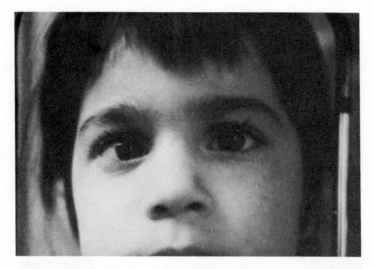

Before

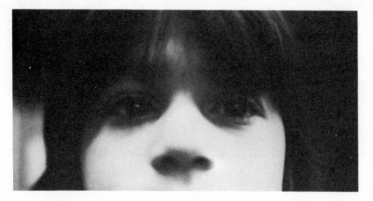

After

Patient 2 At 4 years of age, Rae-Ann demonstrated large esotropia in the right eye which occasionally alternated with the
left eye. Although surgery was suggested, it was rejected by the
child's parents. Following therapy over a three-year period,
interrupted by several vacation breaks due to the very young age
of the patient, a definite reduction of the angle of the eye turn
was achieved. Rae-Ann obtained cosmetic cure.

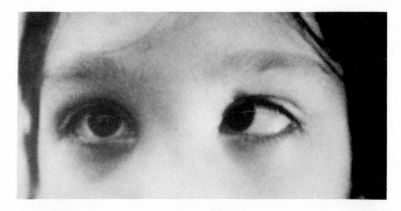

Before

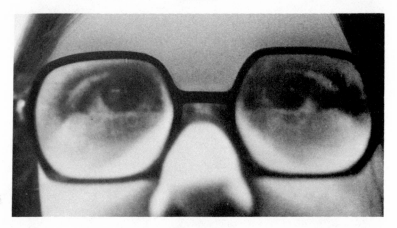

After

Patient 3   Debbie's eyes were first examined when she was two years old. She was slightly far-sighted and suffered from severe esotropia. Wearing eyeglasses somewhat reduced her turning-in eye, however, moderate cosmetic esotropia was still visible. Home orthoptics was prescribed until she was 5¹/₂, at which time optometric vision training was introduced. After 13 months of therapy which actually spanned over a year and a half, due to vacation breaks, the result was a functional, cosmetic cure.

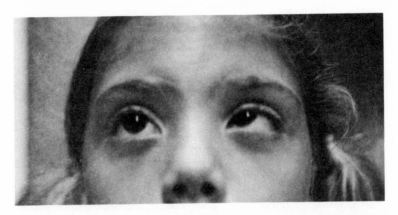

Before

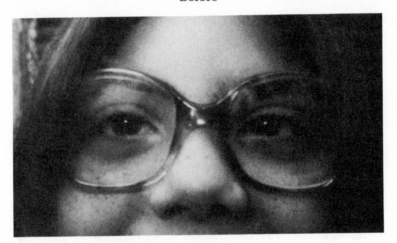

After

Patient 4 Lisa had been seen by various eye surgeons since she was two months old. When she was six years old, paralysis of the muscle which controls the up and down movements of the eyes was discovered. She also turned her eyes in, towards her nose, in an alternate manner. Surgery was recommended, however, due to the paralysis, the chances of success were considered to be very poor. After approximately 1 1/2 years of visual training, Lisa achieved cosmetic cure.

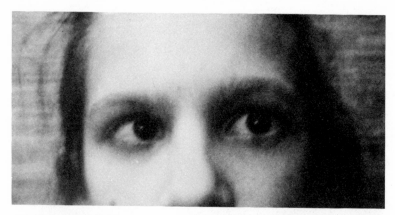

Before

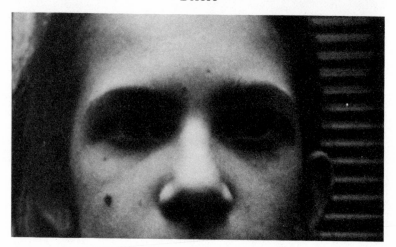

After

Patient 5 Susan had cataracts which were surgically removed
in both eyes. After her operation she developed large esotropia
and surgery was performed for a second time, three years later.
However, the crossed eyes recurred, together with constant
double vision. Susan then underwent optometric vision training
for nine months which straightened her eyes and eliminated the
double vision. She can be considered cosmetically and functionally completely cured.

Although vision therapy takes longer than surgery, it eliminates the risk of an operation and provides the *controlled environment* for learning desired visual skills; by organizing the *total person*, it attempts to re-educate the mind, the body, and the eyes, as it recognizes that vision does not and cannot exist in isolation.

CHAPTER SIXTEEN

THERAPY
AND
TRAINING

WE have emerged out of sight into vision. Vision training or vision therapy is the *re-education* of the visual-motor mode, an extension of visual-motor therapy; it is the process of *learning to see*. "To take you from where you are to where you want to be,"—that's vision training in a nutshell. We want *you* to do the learning and would like to show you how, by taking you out of your present level of visual competency and bringing you forward, step by step, to a new plateau of visual functioning.

When we investigated visual integrity at the University Optometric Center, we asked patients to perform specific tasks. We were interested not so much in *what* they performed but rather in *how* they performed. In this way, we learned how information was processed and whether an individual responded primarily on a *visual*, an *auditory*, or a *tactual* level. We could then gauge each level of visual adequacy and map out a therapy program.

We found that most people fitted in between the clearly visual and the clearly tactual categories; the highly visual type of individual was not too concerned with tactual or auditory clues when completing a specific task; we could therefore start this person on a program of vision therapy geared to a higher visual plane, perhaps involving visual perceptual or visualization procedures.

For an auditory type of individual, we may use a metronome (adjustable clicker) to synthesize audition and vision, and *tap into* the particular functioning of that person. If you can *see* and *hear* something at the same time, a meaningful connection will have been established, and information will be obtained by comparing the data received from two different sense modalities. According to optometrist Dr. Arthur Heinsen, "if, on the other hand, you only see something and, at some later time only, hear it, you don't know what, that you saw sounds like, nor do you know what you heard, looks like." This kind of sensory matching is a fundamental part of any vision training program.

The tactual individual, on the other hand, needs a lower level start, perhaps a tracing exercise, working from *hand leading eye* to *eye leading hand.* We can gradually teach that person to rely less on touch and more on vision. The goal is to free vision from support by lower level perceptual systems, to the extent where vision will eventually become the dominant mode for processing information.

Keep in mind that vision training follows normal developmental principles; you are brought back to the *lowest developmental level* at which proficiency exists and are carried forward through therapy as slowly or as quickly as you are able to progress. Throughout the training, emphasis is on flexibility, rhythm, and timing.

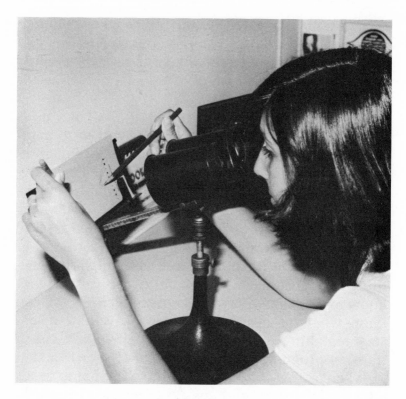

A tracing exercise. From hand leading eye to eye leading hand.

In general, most visual performance problems stem from faulty, early movement patterns; thus training begins at the *gross-motor* stage. It is interesting to note that in a recent study done at the University Optometric Center, 47 per cent of strabismics exhibited poor gross-motor coordination.

In analyzing the more specialized, *fine motor* abilities, we wanted to know whether a child or adult possessed the necessary manipulative and supportive skills expected at a certain age. Can the child tie shoelaces, fasten buttons, use a pen, etc.? *Eye-hand* relationships were next; how efficient were eye-monitoring-hand movements? Does the child need to touch the puzzle before putting it together? At what stage is he in the visual-motor mode? Once these factors were known to us, we could start therapy at the individual's own level. Oculo-motor patterns include all the various eye skills such as focusing, teaming, etc., which we have discussed previously.

Gross- and fine body movement skills are often trained simultaneously with eye movement skills. Clumsy, uncoordinated bodies interact reciprocally with clumsy, uncoordinated eyes. In that case, we might use a balance board and have the patient integrate body balance with eye balance.

Assessing visual judgment is a later, more sophisticated type of therapy. Can you predict and judge size, form, and space? If you can, this ability precedes the highest level of visual function, *problem solving* through *visualization*. For example, when you are asked to predict how many steps it takes to cross a room, we would not expect you to walk across the room but we would expect you to arrive at the answer *visually*.

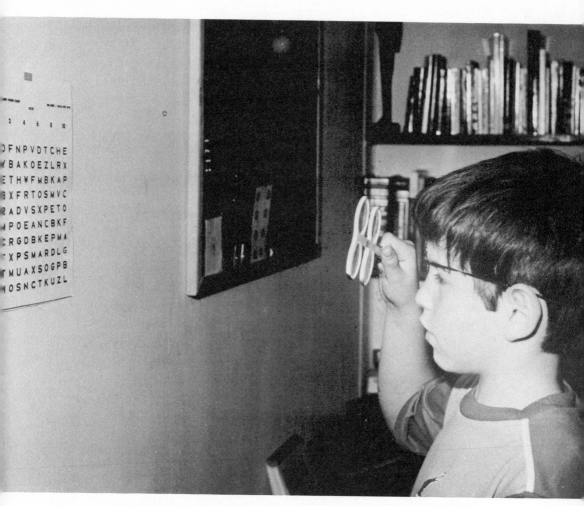

The patient trains through a combination of special lenses which alternately stimulate and relax focusing, to build flexibility into the system.

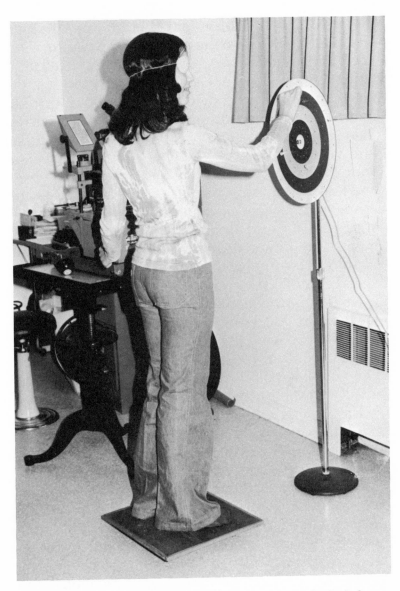

We might put you on a balance board to integrate body balance with eye balance. In this instance, therapy procedure demands using one eye at a time.

In all aspects of visual therapy, ophthalmic lenses and prisms are the unique and powerful tools to be used to achieve visual re-education and rehabilitation as they can alter behavior directly through the visual sense. While psychotherapy employs words to unlock and probe into emotional problems, vision therapy uses lenses and prisms to unlock and probe into visual problems. When we place a lens before your eyes, we alter the input; as a result, the object you look at may appear to have moved in space and changed in size, even though it remains stationary. We can also cause an object to appear one hundred miles away, although you can still touch it with your hand! The creation of this sensory mismatch sets up a visual conflict. How you deal with this conflict tells us, in fact, how dependent you are on either vision or touch. Can you still operate visually through the lens? Do you need the reinforcement of your tactual sense to confirm where the object really is in space? Can you make it all fit together?

By working your way through various types of lenses, you gain practice and become flexible, moving and visually guiding yourself through new space. You recapitulate early, spontaneous learning and re-live previous, sensory movement experiences.

According to optometrist Dr. Lawrence Macdonald, "optometric visual training involves rematching the visual and kinesthetic co-ordinates. As the kinesthetic system begins to re-adjust, old memories and experiences may surface to the conscious level. Some of these may be loaded with emotional content." In his excellent article, "Implications of Critical Empathy, Primal Scream and Identity Crisis in

Optometric Visual Therapy," Dr. Macdonald goes on to point out that at a certain stage of vision therapy, the stage he calls "critical" or "breakthrough time," optometrists have observed a curious response which seems to have its counterpart in psychotherapy.

At this time, the patient first comes to terms with his visual space world. A simultaneous release of pent-up, emotional energy that accompanied previous associations and half-forgotten memories occurs, resulting in sobbing, crying, and general disorientation.

In vision therapy this is when the patient is asked: "What are you aware of feeling?" or "be aware of feeling something." According to Dr. Macdonald, typical answers would be: "I cannot look and think at the same time; I simply must close my eyes to get myself together; I feel that my body is anchored on one side and will not move, as if someone or something were holding me; I cannot get away!"

Some of the fears and anxieties experienced during vision therapy are difficult to describe. Patients gain a certain insight into things and reach a level of understanding not otherwise possible, nor normally within their grasp. They become more confident and can operate more efficiently in their environment, however artificial it may be.

Our contemporary culture and the artificial environment we live in has stifled sensory pleasures, pleasures felt and enjoyed at an earlier age. Aldous Huxley states in *The Doors of Perception*, that with mescalin, an hallucinogen, "visual impressions are greatly intensified and the eye recovers some of the perceptual innocence of childhood, when the sensum

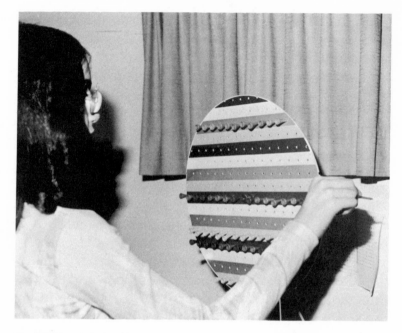

By using a special prismatic lens, we are creating a sensory mismatch, to find out whether the patient can still operate visually through the lens.

was not immediately and automatically subordinated to the concept." Vision therapy, through the recapitulation of early, sensory movement experiences, alters consciousness in a similar way and can be as powerful as any drug in obtaining pleasure and avoiding pain.

The ultimate goal of vision therapy is to enhance our ability to *think visually*. On the concrete level, almost every area of practical creativity calls for some kind of visualizing and the ability to manipulate, recall, and reproduce visual patterns. The best performance by an athlete, an architect, a dancer, or a surgeon is invariably preceded by the *visual picture* of the desired action. On the abstract level, vision therapy presents the unique opportunity to alter consciousness in a positive direction, to free us from cultural and environmental limitations, and to allow us to develop new dimensions of thought.

As you transcend the need for conscious observation, visual-motor therapy hopes to take you out of the commonplace level of SIGHT into a new awareness, where seeing and doing, perceiving and reacting, sensory reception and motor expression become an almost simultaneous experience. VISION can then become the ultimate sensory experience, beyond which lie the new and extraordinary realities we constantly seek to discover.

APPENDIX

EDUCATOR'S CHECKLIST
OBSERVABLE CLUES TO CLASSROOM VISION PROBLEMS

PREPARED BY:
Section on Children's Vision Care and Guidance
Optometric Extension Program Foundation, Inc.
(A Nonprofit, Tax-exempt Foundation for Education
and Research in Vision)
Duncan, Oklahoma 73533

Student's
Name _____ Date _____

1. APPEARANCE OF EYES:
   One eye turns in or out at any time _____
   Reddened eyes or lids _____
   Eyes tear excessively _____
   Encrusted eyelids _____
   Frequent styes on lids _____

2. COMPLAINTS WHEN USING EYES AT DESK:
   Headaches in forehead or temples _____
   Burning or itching after reading or desk work _____
   Nausea or dizziness _____
   Print blurs after reading a short time _____

3. BEHAVIORAL SIGNS OF VISUAL PROBLEMS:

   A. *Eye Movement Abilities (Ocular Motility)*

      Head turns as reads across page   _____

      Loses place often during reading   _____

      Needs finger or marker to keep place _____

      Displays short attention span in reading or copying _____

      Too frequently omits words _____

      Repeatedly omits "small" words _____

      Writes up or down hill on paper _____

      Rereads or skips lines unknowingly _____

      Orients drawings poorly on page _____

   B. *Eye Teaming Abilities (Binocularity)*

      Complains of seeing double (diplopia) _____

      Repeats letters within words _____

      Omits letters, numbers or phrases _____

      Misaligns digits in number columns _____

      Squints, closes or covers one eye _____

      Tilts head extremely while working at desk _____

      Consistently shows gross postural deviations at all desk activities _____

   C. *Eye-Hand Coordination Abilities*

      Must feel things to assist in any interpretation required _____

      Eyes not used to "steer" hand movements (extreme lack of orientation, placement of words or drawings on page) _____

      Writes crookedly, poorly spaced: cannot stay on ruled lines _____

Misaligns both horizontal and vertical
series of numbers   _____

Uses his hand or fingers to keep his
place on the page   _____

Uses other hand as "spacer" to control
spacing and alignment on page   _____

Repeatedly confuses left-right
directions   _____

D. *Visual Form Perception (Visual
Comparison, Visual Imagery,
Visualization)*

Mistakes words with same or similar
beginnings   _____

Fails to recognize same word in next
sentence   _____

Reverses letters and/or words in
writing and copying   _____

Confuses likenesses and minor
differences   _____

Confuses same word in same sentence   _____

Repeatedly confuses similar
beginnings and endings of words   _____

Fails to visualize what is read either
silently or orally   _____

Whispers to self for reinforcement
while reading silently   _____

Returns to "drawing with fingers" to
decide likes and differences   _____

E. *Refractive Status (Near-sightedness,
Far-sightedness, Focus Problems, etc.)*

Comprehension reduces as reading
continued; loses interest too quickly   _____

Mispronounces similar words as
continues reading   _____

Blinks excessively at desk tasks
and/or reading; not elsewhere _____

Holds book too closely; face too close
to desk surface _____

Avoids all possible near-centered
tasks _____

Complains of discomfort in tasks that
demand visual interpretation _____

Closes or covers one eye when reading
or doing desk work _____

Makes errors in copying from
chalkboard to paper on desk _____

Makes errors in copying from
reference book to notebook _____

Squints to see chalkboard, or requests
to move nearer _____

Rubs eyes during or after short periods
of visual activity _____

Fatigues easily; blinks to make
chalkboard clear up after desk task _____

OBSERVER'S SUGGESTIONS:

Signed _____

(Encircle): Teacher; Nurse; Remedial Teacher; Psychologist;
Vision Consultant; Other.

INDEX

Full spectrum,
  fluorescent bulb, *94*
  natural light, *93*
  plastic lens, *95*
  plastic, neutral gray sunlenses, *92, 93*
  plastic windows, *94*
Fusion, *31, 33*
  test of, *33, 34, inside jacket*

G
Glaucoma, *43*
Greenwald, I., *164*
Gross-motor stage (*see Movement*)

H
Harmon, Darell B., *15, 66, 67, 84-86, 132, 137-141*
Harmon distance, *133, 134*
Heliotropic organism, *79*
High visual type (*see Vision Therapy and Training*)
Huxley, Aldous, *179*

I
Ilg, Frances, *121*

K
Kephart, Newell C., *21*
Kirlian photography, *83*

L
Lazy eye, *53*
  amblyopia, *53*
  syndrome, *112*
Learning disabled, *68*
Lens,
  bifocal, *51*
  dual-focus, *51*
  near, *14, 15*
  negative, *14*
  ophthalmic, *178*